Intermittent Fasting for Women Over 50

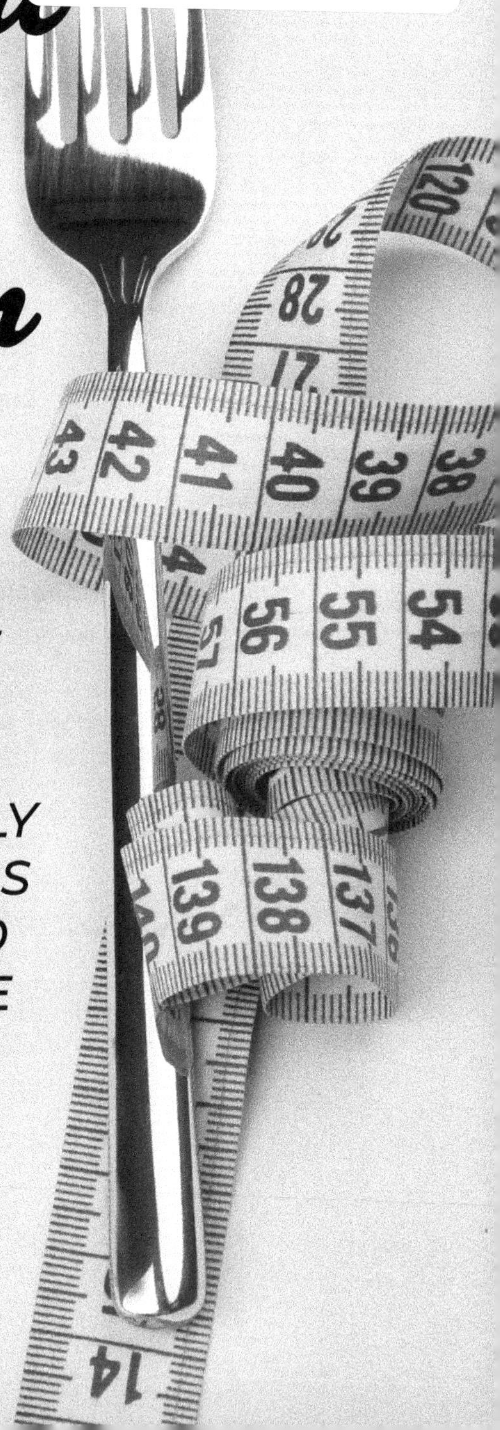

THE WINNING FORMULA TO LOSE WEIGHT, UNLOCK METABOLISM AND REJUVENATE. IT ONLY TAKES A FEW HOURS WITHOUT FOOD TO OBTAIN IMMEDIATE RESULTS.

TABLE OF CONTENTS

Introduction

Over the age of 50, it is increasingly difficult for a woman to lose weight and we are obsessed with those extra pounds that accumulate in areas where we do not want them to, such as hips and love handles. Intermittent fasting is an alternative to the usual diet, and can also become a way of life, if you think of the countless benefits that calorie restriction brings to body and mind.

The different types of intermittent fasting allow us to evaluate and choose the most suitable one for us, adapting it to our needs and lifestyle.

Obviously, it is necessary to maintain a balanced and healthy diet, rich in vegetables and whole grains and that provides all the macronutrients needed by the body, as well as the right amount of fat (preferably vegetable) and avoid junk food, seasoned and too salty. All in all, however, you can eat anything, even taking a few whims from time to time.

Fasting has positive implications for the health of women over 50. Science has shown that reducing calorie intake prolongs life, because it acts on the metabolic function of longevity genes, reduces senile diseases, cancer, cardiovascular diseases and neurodegenerative ones such as Alzheimer's and Parkinson's disease. In addition, especially for women over 50, it has multiple benefits on mood, fights depression, contributes to the improvement of energy, libido and concentration. And as if that weren't enough, it gives the skin a better look.

To start this type of "diet" you must first of all be in good health and in any case, before starting, it is always better to consult your doctor. The female body is particularly sensitive to calorie restriction, because the hypothalamus, a gland in the brain responsible for the production of hormones, is stimulated. These hormones risk going haywire with a drastic reduction in calories or too long a fast. The advice is therefore to start gradually, perhaps introducing some vegetable snacks during fasting hours (fennel, lettuce, endive, radicchio).

As mentioned, in women, intermittent fasting works differently than in men. Sometimes it is more difficult for women to get results. Physiological and weight benefits are still possible, but sometimes require a different approach. In addition, intermittent fasting on non-consecutive days is better able to keep those annoying hormones under control. Various scientific evidence shows that in order to achieve fat loss, fasting must be tailored to the sex.

Fasting, after all, represents the easiest and at the same time powerful detoxification and regeneration therapy that we can offer to cells and the whole organism. Putting certain functions at physiological rest does not, in fact, mean that organs and tissues go into stand-by. On the contrary, thanks to the absence of a continuous metabolic commitment, they can dedicate themselves to something else, activating all those processes of self-repair, catabolism, excretion and cell turnover that only in the absence of nutrients can take place at the highest levels.

Because health, diet, reproductivity, and nutritional needs are all altered for mature and menopausal women, their relationships with intermittent fasting can be very different from young women's. For instance, while young women ought to be careful about how intermittent fasting can affect their fertility levels, older women can practice intermittent fasting freely without these concerns. Therefore, more mature women can apply the weight-loss techniques of intermittent fasting to their lives (and waistlines) without the worry of what negative side-effects might arise in the future.

For menopausal women, however, the situation is a little bit different than it is for fully mature women. People going through menopause have to deal with daily hormone fluctuations that cause hot and cold flashes, sleeplessness, anxiety, irregular periods, and more. At the beginning of this process, intermittent fasting will not necessarily help, and it could even make your situation more stressful.

For women in this situation who are actively going through menopause, you must remember that your body is extremely sensitive to changes right now. If you do find that intermittent fasting helps and that short periods of fast are effective, you must also make sure to increase the intensity of your fast as gradually as possible so your body can adjust without creating horrible hormonal repercussions for yourself and everyone around you. For the fully mature woman, intermittent fasting will not make you as cranky, moody, irregular in the period, or otherwise because those hormones won't be affecting you at all anymore, or at least, hardly at all. Your dietary and eating schedule choices become more liberated from the effects they used to have on your hormonal health as the years go by. Therefore, if you're seeking weight loss, better energy, a physiological jolt back to health, or what have you, try out IF without concern and see what happens. For these types of women, intermittent fasting is set to provide hope through eased depression, the lessened likelihood of cancer (or its recurrence), promised weight loss, and more

Chapter 01

The Magical Diet of Intermittent Fasting at 50. Why Try It

Being a woman is one thing. Being a woman over the age of 50 is another. With age slowly creeping in on you, your body begins to experience some changes. If you are self-aware and alert, you will notice these changes early enough. If you aren't, however, it will likely take a while.

At age 50 and over, it naturally becomes more challenging to shed weight. This is because metabolism will decrease, joints might be more prone to ache, muscle mass will decrease, and you might even experience sleep issues. In addition to these, you'll become more at risk of developing certain age-related diseases and health conditions.

Some of the changes your body might be subtle, but they are nonetheless veiled threats to a fully functional body system and definitely to the longevity we all seek.

This is why it is imperative to seek out measures, lifestyles, and diets that could help you lose fat, especially dangerous belly fat. Losing fat will drastically reduce the risks of developing health issues, such as diabetes, heart attack, and cancer.

Below are a few reasons you need to consider intermittent fasting seriously:

Weight Loss

A very high percentage of people who are currently into intermittent fasting did so because they either want to guard against piling up excess body fat or because they want to lose weight. That makes weight loss a primary reason women over the age of 50 should consider giving intermittent fasting a try.

Intermittent fasting generally helps boost metabolism in the body by promoting thermogenesis or production of heat. This will lead to excess body fat being burned and used to fuel the body's activities.

Another way intermittent fasting can help solve weight is by reducing hunger. Thus, the stomach will always have the illusion of being filled.

Weight loss becomes even more natural when the keto diet is combined with intermittent fasting. They both complement each other.

Muscle and Joint Health

Research efforts also proved that intermittent fasting could help women over 50 to improve their muscle and joint health. Some of the researchers discovered that the fasting period affects the way the body produces hormones. This will help strengthen the bones and forestall against things like arthritic symptoms and lower back pain.

Intermittent Fasting Can Help To Prevent Cancer

Women over 50 are at risk of developing some kinds of cancer. Intermittent fasting, as shown in research, can cut off some of the pathways leading to cancer. Intermittent fasting can also help slow down the rate at which an existing tumor grows in the body.

Intermittent Fasting and Mental Health

Because of the changes in the body, the hormonal imbalance and the uncertainty surrounding the state of things, it could be a mentally disturbing period for women over 50.

A 2018 study showed that women who practiced intermittent fasting reported improvement in moods and self-esteem while anxiety and depression levels dropped.

If you are prone to depression and anxiety disorders, intermittent fasting might just be the easiest way out. But you have to speak with your medical professional first.

Intermittent Fasting Helps with Sleep and Clarity

Hormonal changes in the body can cause one's sleeping pattern to be destabilized, especially around the post-menstrual age.

It is soothing to discover that many older women have testified about how the intermittent fasting lifestyle has improved their sleeping pattern.

If you're currently experiencing sleep issues, intermittent fasting is definitely an option for you.

Intermittent Fasting and Longevity

Perhaps the greatest bane of growing older is that old age opens up the body to more risk of developing diseases.

Ultimately, intermittent fasting became so popular among women aged 50 and older because of how it evidently helps them live longer and in good health.

Some even say it was tailor-made for older women.

Intermittent Fasting Boosts Productivity

Growing old can be quite a boring stage of life for people struggling with their health each day. It could rob them of the joy of living, experiencing life, and getting things done.

Older people are happier when they can stay fit and healthy. While it might be retirement age, there are a lot of things you might want to do with your life at that point, activities that could bring you fulfilment if you're healthy enough to partake in them.

Intermittent fasting helps you experience a boost in productivity by helping to keep you fit and in good health.

In summary, intermittent fasting is the answer to many of the adverse effects of growing older. It keeps you in charge of your body and teaches you how to get the best out of your body system, effectively maximizing your potential to remain in good health for as long as possible.
Ensure that you pick the right fasting method. You might need to pair it with a diet, keto probably. You would also need to discuss this with your doctor/dietitian/psychologist to ascertain what is truly right for you and what is not. Women over 50 cannot afford to take certain health risks. So you have to be sure you can trust your health and wellness regime.

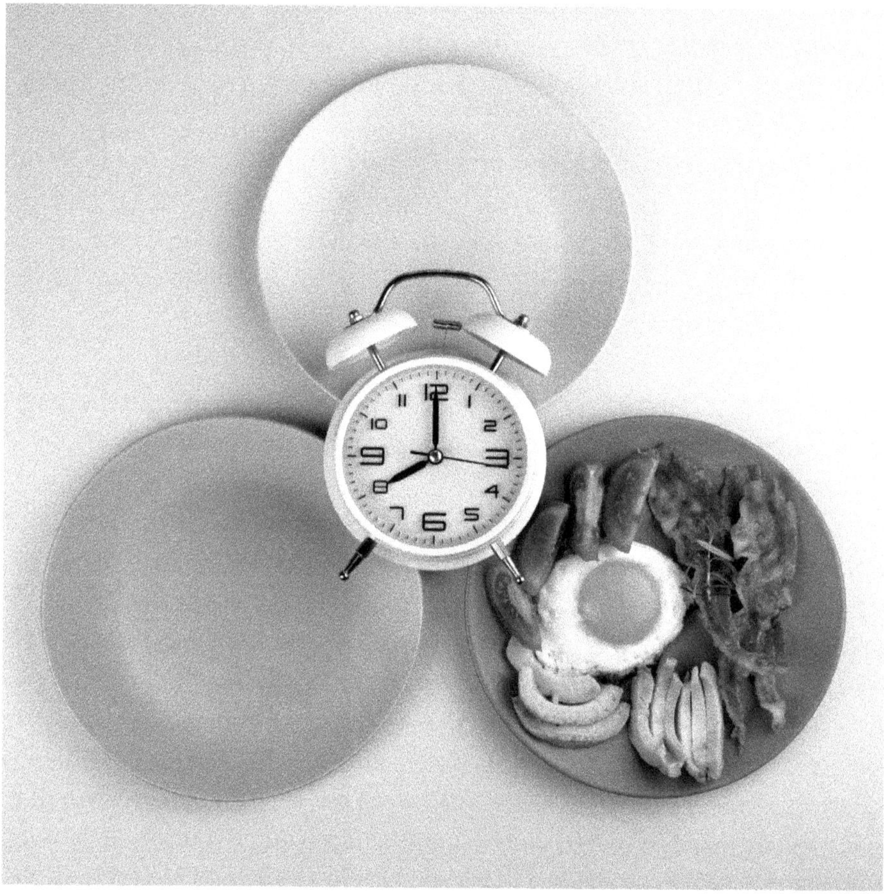

Chapter 02

Benefits of Intermittent Fasting

Until now, you must have realized that intermittent fasting is simply switching between fasting and eating. Eating is done in cycles or specific periods and fasting is followed after.

Anti-Aging Effect.

Intermittent fasting has been proved to regulate hormones and aid in anti-aging effects. This will be natural since your body will have weight loss, more activity and hormonal balance.

Helpful Hormonal Behavior.

The reason why this needs to be talked about is because many ladies develop hormonal problems after age fifty or around it. First, let me start with some general advantages. When you adapt your body to intermittent fasting, the body undergoes several hormonal changes.

1. *Reduction in insulin levels happens because of intermittent fasting. This reduction of insulin leads to fast metabolism along with fat burning. The reduction*

in insulin is also vital since its imbalance can be a serious problem in women above fifty.

2. *For females who experience muscle pain after the age of fifty or around it, the intermittent fasting is something profoundly effective. The human growth hormone that is responsible for muscle gain is sped up by the process of intermittent fasting. It is relieving for people who have muscular pain. For females above fifty, arthritis is usually common. The intermittent fasting can help you relieve the pain by enhancing muscle growth along with bone healing.*
3. *The fat storing and hunger hormones benefit quite a lot from the intermittent fasting. The hormones responsible for blood sugar control, hunger improvement and metabolism are affected in a positive way. Especially for females who have blood sugar problems, the intermittent fasting can prove to be quite something useful. It has low insulin resistance and increased metabolism. I would recommend using intermittent fasting along with supervision of a doctor as medical way to solve your blood sugar problem. Since the low insulin resistance and faster metabolism is used to control the blood sugar, it is imperative that you are monitoring your glucose levels.*
4. *There are other negative sides to hormonal imbalance which can lead to increased hunger. Intermittent fasting comes to the rescue here! Some critics claim that intermittent fasting will leave you in a starved state. However, this is far from truth. The intermittent fasting*

method actually improves the hunger hormones, causing your body to crave less and less in comparison to before.

5. *Women have a part of the brain that is responsible for communicating between ovaries and the brain. When that part doesn't work well, the fertility problems can occur. Here, I would recommend the usage of proper intermittent fasting. If it is not done properly here, it can mess up your hormones and cause imbalance instead. However, this doesn't mean intermittent fasting doesn't give benefit in this state. The intermittent fasting if done two days a week can actually give relief. (You will need to consult a doctor about it).*
6. *The hormones that protect against the disease are naturally strengthened. This actually helps in scenarios especially for women above fifty. The immune system can be strengthened that actually helps a lot.*

Reduction in Weight.

There are many reasons why intermittent fasting helps in reduction of weight. However, I will be discussing two situations here. The first one will be applicable to general health fitness issues. The second situation is specifically for women above fifty. It is related to weight gain after menopause hits.

Generally, many females get into the intermittent fasting because they want to lose their weight. This is first advantage of it since intermittent fasting will lead to consumption of lesser meals than before. This will also allow a lower intake of calories. Several of the hormones that I listed above are involved in fat burning and it is facilitated a lot in intermittent fasting. The body fat is naturally broken down and it is consumed in a natural process. Fat burning is further enhanced by the metabolism. The weight loss is thus a direct effect of intermittent fasting.

However, for females around the age of fifty, there is another problem that usually occurs. Since this is a female specific book, the information that I am about to provide is quite open.

Menopause occurs when the menstrual cycle ends. Usually in aged females, menopause occurs when you have gone twelve months without menstrual period. The age of women that get affected by it is around 40s, but it is also around 50s. It is a natural biological process. Yet, it is not an easy process. The physical symptoms are quite common. Hot flashes are the most common physical symptoms. This also may disrupt your sleep, causing the tiredness. It is really not a pretty situation especially if you are a working lady in her fifties. Even if you are a housewife, this can present problems. Your overall energy will be lowered. Apart from that, it is not uncommon for women undergoing menopause to show emotional issues. There are many treatments available for the issues arising from this natural process. One of the most effective methods for menopause treatment is intermittent fasting.

Usually, the menopause is followed by following symptoms,

1. *Irregular periods*
2. *Vaginal Dryness*
3. *Hot flashes (can become uncomfortable particularly in summers)*
4. *Chills*
5. *Night sweats*
6. *Sleep problems*
7. *Mood changes (the kid throwing tantrums may make you want to smack him)*
8. *Weight gain and slowed metabolism*
9. *Thinning hair and dry skin*
10. *Loss of breast fullness*

One of the most common problems after menopause is unexpected pounds which you might have suddenly put up. Why would that happen? That happens because the metabolism during menopause becomes increasingly slow. This may lead to weight gain that may come off as unex-

pected during this natural biological process. This can also come with low sensitivity to insulin that will end up messing up the sugar and carbohydrates digestion. All of this leads to weight gain too. It may lead to depression for some ladies. The body is starting to act in strangest manner, and you don't know how to control it. There are methods for easing the process. I have personally seen first-hand the benefits of chamomile tea. The weight gain aspect of menopause can cause anxiety and depression.

The intermittent fasting will definitely help you in the weight loss that you aim for. I am not going to sugar-coat it. It is a process that may require dedication, but you will end up getting its benefits.

Lowering Resistance of Insulin.

The lowering of insulin resistance simply can lead to avoidance of type 2 diabetes. Some of the women over fifty actually have problem with blood sugar levels. Some of them have issues with diabetes and intermittent fasting helps in that. Anything that helps with insulin reduction helps in protection against sugar level imbalance. This will end up creating protection against type 2 diabetes. In some cases, scientific studies showed that the intermittent fasting was particularly effective against the kidney damage which is caused by a severe form of diabetes. It is thus an excellent method for type 2 diabetes prevention.

Reduction in Oxidative Stress.

The oxidative stress is responsible for many issues in your body. It is responsible for many chronic diseases. The reason behind it is because it is responsible for introducing unstable molecules in your body. They interact with other molecules and end up damaging them too. This can lead to huge increase in chronic disease rate. It is something that the women over fifty should be vary of.

Intermittent fasting has shown to be quite effective in this scenario. The oxidative stress is substantially reduced in case of intermittent fasting. Furthermore, the inflammation is also reduced by intermittent fasting that is another driver of all diseases. Thus, the intermittent fasting is quite a useful technique in this scenario especially for women.

Heart Health.

The heart health is one of the most sensitive issues that require caretaking. When one reaches above, it is imperative that cholesterol is checked. The increase in cholesterol can very easily lead to heart diseases and in severe cases, heart attack. When one does intermittent fasting, this leads to lower calorie intake. This will in turn, lead to lesser choles-

terol. Henceforth, this leads to better heart health. Research is still being done on this aspect, but generally intermittent fasting has been proved to improve heart health.

Cell Repair.

Over the time, our body accumulates waste proteins that serve no function. The process of intermittent fasting ends up producing a process called autophagy which initiates cell breakdown. The cell breaks down ends up removing all waste products and proteins that serve no function. This automatically cleans up the body.

This process of cleaning up gives way for new cells to be produced. The production of new cells without the need to take in any medication or supplement is a blessing at the age of fifty or beyond. Nudging the biological process this way to act in a healthy manner will end up giving you much better health than usual.

Enhanced Mental Capability.

Mental capability is something that decreases with time and age. At the age of fifty or beyond, it is imperative that body's natural processes are enhanced. Some women use medicines or supplements to do it. However, these things usually end up producing hormonal imbalance by messing up by some of already present hormones in the body. That would not be such a good thing. Taking pills for depression and anxiety is really not preferred for aged women.

Mental capability is one of the things that also increase with the practice of intermittent fasting. The intermittent fasting increases the levels of a brain hormone. This brain hormone becomes deficient in depression. When this hormone is produced properly, the mental capacity increases.

Curing Cancer.

Fasting has been proved to improve the metabolism. Some of these effects are directly correlated to the reduction of cancer risk. Though much research has been done and still needs to be done, the fasting has somewhat a positive relation to the reduction of cancer. Intermittent fasting is no different. It may actually be possible with intermittent fasting to improve immunity and henceforth, aid cancer prevention.

Prevention Against Alzheimer's Disease.

There is currently no cure for Alzheimer's disease. Therefore, to prevent it is something that is quite feasible and only possible solution. With intermittent fasting being your lifestyle, the disease can be prevented. Intermittent fasting can very easily lead to brain function enhancement.

The intermittent fasting also leads to increase in helpful hormones that reduce the chances of Alzheimer's disease. Much research needs to be done on this aspect though.

Chapter 03

Meal Plan for 14 Days

The intermittent fasting diet helps you lose weight quickly because it speeds up your metabolism. It is based on alternating full and regular meals with fasting during the hours of the day.

But what to eat in the fed stages of the various diets of intermittent fasting? Following a meal plan is highly essential if you want to lose weight. When you combine your meal plans with intermittent fasting, you will begin to see massive results. Women above 50 need to keep track of their meals as they face the reality of gaining weight easier than losing it.

Meal Plan Week 1

Days	Breakfast	Snack	Lunch	Snack	Dinner
Monday	One large grapefruit and 3 Scrambled Eggs	25 almonds	One apple Turkey Wrap	A piece of string cheese	Spicy Chicken with Side salad, dressing with two tablespoons of olive oil or vinegar

Days	Breakfast	Snack	Lunch	Snack	Dinner
Tuesday	One large grapefruit, ham, and Lean Eggs	25 almonds	One apple, Cheese Burrito, and Black Bean	A piece of string cheese	Bun and Veggie Burger together with a salad dressed with four tablespoons of olive oil or vinegar, and finally one serving of sweet potato fries

Days	Breakfast	Snack	Lunch	Snack	Dinner
Wednesday	Zero-fat Greek yogurt and Berry Wafflewich	Two tablespoons of hummus and 15 snap peas	One apple and Gobleguac Sandwich	One piece of string cheese and banana	Two cups of broccoli, One cup of brown rice, and Steamed Snapper together with Pesto
Thursday	One large grapefruit and zero-fat Greek yogurt	One Luna Bar	25 almonds and the I-Am-Not-Eating-Salad Salad	Four tablespoons of hummus and 30 baby carrots	Two cups of snow peas, a cup of brown rice and Chicken Spinach Parm

Days	Breakfast	Snack	Lunch	Snack	Dinner
Friday	One banana and Loaded Vegetable Omelet	One piece of string cheese	One apple and a Turkey Wrap	Two tablespoons of hummus and ten cherry tomatoes	Two cups of broccoli, rice with Quick Lemon Chicken
Saturday	One large grapefruit and three Scrambled Eggs	25 almonds	Leftover cups of broccoli, Chicken Marengo and Penne	Zero-fat Greek yogurt and piece of string cheese	Two cups of snow peas and Thai Beef Lettuce Wraps
Sunday	One banana and Loaded Vegetable Omelet	Zero-fat Greek yogurt and piece of string cheese	One apple and the I-Am-Not-Eating-Salad Salad	One Luna Bar and teen cherry tomatoes	One cup of brown rice, 2 cups of broccoli and Tofu Stir-Fry

Meal Plan Week 2

Days	Breakfast	Snack	Lunch	Snack	Dinner
Monday	One large grapefruit and 3 Scrambled Eggs	25 almonds and zero-fat Greek yogurt	Leftover one cup of brown rice and Tofu Stir-Fry	One piece of string cheese and banana	Two cups of broccoli, rice, and Quick Lemon Chicken
Tuesday	One banana and Giant Omelet Scramble	Two small boxes of raisins	One apple and Turkey Wrap	One Lärabar	Two cups of broccoli, one cup of brown rice and Grilled Cilantro-Lime Chicken

Days	Breakfast	Snack	Lunch	Snack	Dinner
Wednesday	One large grapefruit and Loaded Vegetable Omelet	One banana and Zero fat Greek yogurt	One apple and Turkey Wrap	Two tablespoons of hummus and 15 baby carrots	One cup of brown rice, two cups of broccoli and Steamed Snapper with
Thursday	One medium grapefruit, ham, and Lean Eggs	25 almonds and a piece of string cheese	One apple and Mediterranean Hummus Wrap	Mini bag and Smart Balance Light Butter Popcorn	Two cups of broccoli, chicken Marengo with Penne
Friday	One large grapefruit and Don't-Get-Fat French toast	One piece of string cheese and small boxes of raisins	One apple and the I-Am-Not-Eating-Salad Salad	15 baby carrots and 2 Tbsp of hummus	Salad and Miso Salmon and Two tablespoons of olive oil dressing

Days	Breakfast	Snack	Lunch	Snack	Dinner
Saturday	One large grapefruit and Loaded Vegetable Omelet	Mini bag of Smart Balance Light Butter Popcorn	One apple and Mediterranean Hummus Wrap	Zero-fat Greek yogurt	Two cups of broccoli, vegetables, and Whole Wheat Pasta
Sunday	One large grapefruit and Giant Omelet Scramble	One piece of string cheese	Leftover Vegetables with Whole Wheat Pasta and one apple	25 almonds	One cup of brown rice and Tofu Stir-Fry

Chapter 04

Intermittent Fasting and Supplements

Not all supplements can provide the health benefits you need. Taking the wrong supplements, especially while you are on intermittent fasting, may bring harm. The right types of health supplements can significantly boost the effects of intermittent fasting.

We will briefly discuss the problems with taking generic supplements, how to choose the right health supplements for those who are into intermittent fasting, and a comprehensive list of health supplements that you should take.

The Problem with Multivitamins

Multivitamins are very popular. Millions of people around the world are taking multivitamins, so people think that they are indispensable for fighting disease and malnutrition. This is, in fact, a misconception. In reality, not everyone can benefit from multivitamins and instead choose targeted supplements.

Nutritional Imbalance

Many multivitamins contain too much of specific nutrients such as Vitamin A or C, and not enough of the other essential nutrients such as magnesium. So there is a tendency to overdose on few nutrients and not taking enough of the others.

Some manufacturers still include a long list of multivitamins on their labels, but the truth is, some of these vitamins are in very small amounts. Many consumers ignore the insubstantial amounts of important nutrients. How can you fit a range of nutrients in only one pill? Also, we need to consider the nutritional needs of each person. A bodybuilder will require a different set of nutrients compared to a lactating mom.

Low Quality of Multivitamins

Each type of nutrient behaves differently inside the body. While folate is an important B vitamin, folic acid - the form found in generic multivitamins, may increase the risk of colon cancer according to a study published by the University of Chile.

This could be the reason why some researches such as a 2009 study published by the University of East Finland sug-

gest a connection between multivitamins and increase in mortality, while another research commissioned by the American Medical Association in 2009 reveals no benefit in taking multivitamins.

Furthermore, many multivitamins are manufactured with additives and fillers, which make it difficult for the body to absorb nutrients. Therefore, a minimal amount of important nutrients may reach your cells.

We are actually getting what we pay for with multivitamins. You may convince yourself and choose the generic multivitamins in the store, or you may add a bit and actually choose targeted supplements to help improve your health.

Supplements and Fasting

Eating whole and natural foods are still the best source to get the important nutrients that our body needs. Remember, whole foods may behave differently from their individual components. For example, the nutrients from a piece of broccoli are more accessible compared to consuming the equal amount of nutrients from a powder or a pill.

The antioxidants sourced from natural foods are beneficial, but consuming mega doses of some synthetic antioxidants may come with risks such as the growth of tumor based on a 1993 toxicology research from the University of Hamburg.

Food synergy enables the nutrients in food to work together. Hence, food is more powerful compared to its components. This is why it is crucial to begin with a diet that is rich in nutrients, then add supplements that are based on your goals and needs.

It is important to take note that just because something is natural doesn't mean it is helpful. There is a tendency for some, especially the health buffs, to abuse even food based vitamins and herbal supplements.

These supplements are still vulnerable from contaminants and heavy metals from manufacturing. Be sure to check the sourcing and quality testing of your supplements. It is ideal to check with a licensed professional who can recommend safe brands of supplements.

Chapter 05

Other Tips To Follow To Make It More Effective

Intermittent fasting is not easy. We need support as much as possible and anything that can make your journey easier. Below are some of the tips that will make your journey smooth and effective.

Decide on your fasting window.

Intermittent fasting is not a strict time-based diet. This means that you can choose the number of hours to fast and when to fast either day or night. The fasting and eating window periods are not a must to be the same every day.

Ensure you get enough sleep.

When you get enough sleep, you become healthier, and your overall well-being is guaranteed. When we sleep, the body operates certain functions in the body that helps burn calories and improves the metabolic rate.

Eat healthy Avoid eating anything you want after a fast.

Healthy meals should be your focus. They will help you get the required nutrients like vitamins, which will give you more energy during the fasting period.

Drink more water.

One of the best decisions you can make during a fast is to drink water. It will keep your body hydrated and taking water before meals can significantly reduce appetite.

Start small.

If you have never tried it before, there is no way you start fasting and go for a whole 48 hours without a meal. For beginners, you can start by having your food at 8 pm, for example, and having nothing again until 8 am the next day. It will be easier since sleep is incorporated in your eating window.

Avoid stress.

Intermittent might be hard to do if you are stressed. This is because stress can trigger an overindulgence of food to some people. It is also easier to feed on junk when stressed to feel better. That's why when on intermittent fasting, you are advised to avoid if not control your stress levels.

Be disciplined.

Remember that fasting means the abstinence of food until a particular time. When fasting, be true to yourself and avoid eating before the stipulated time. It will ensure that you lose maximum weight and benefit health-wise from intermittent fasting.

Keep off flavored drinks.

Most flavored drink says that they are low in sugar, but in the real sense, they are not. Flavored drinks contain artificial sweeteners, which will affect your health negatively. They will also increase your appetite, causing you to overeat, and this will make you gain weight instead of losing.

Find something to do when fasting.

It is said that an idle mind is the devil's workshop. When you are on intermittent fasting and not busy, you will be thinking about food, and this will make you break your fast before the stipulated time. You can keep yourself busy by running errands, listening to music, or even taking a walk in the park.

Exercising.

Exercise can be done when fasting, but it is not a must. Mild exercises can be done even at home. By exercising, you will build your muscle strength, and your body fat will burn faster.

Chapter 06

The Intermittent Fasting Types

There are various ways you could engage in intermittent fasting. These types have been proven to give the same effects that have made people start fasting, and some of these potentials benefits include the loss of weight and fat. Some have also discovered that it helps in reducing the risk of getting some diseases.

These are some of the types that are popular and have been proven to show effectiveness:

The 16/8 Method

This involves fasting for a total period of 16 hours in the 24 hours that makes a day.

This method requires a daily fast of 14 hours for women and 16 hours for men. You'll have to limit the times you eat to a total of 8- to 10-hour eating window. With this method, you can incorporate 2 to 3 or more meals in a day.

Martin Berkhan, the famous fitness expert, made this method popular. Some refer to it as the Leangains protocol. It is the most widely known because it is almost natural.

The hours you skip meals fall under the time you are either sleeping or working. Most people who skip their breakfast and finish dinner before eight are actually doing the 16-hour protocol, but they don't know that.

Women are instructed to fast for 14 to 15 hours because most do better with this short range, and during the fast you have to eat healthy foods during the eating window. The results you want to achieve won't be forthcoming if there's a lot of junk in your food.

You can take water and coffee during the fasting hours as well as other drinks that are noncaloric.

To fast with this method, your last meal should be by 8 p.m. while your first meal should be by 12 p.m.

The 5.2 Diet

British journalist Michael Mosley popularized this method. It has also been called the fast diet.

This method requires that you limit the number of calories you consume to only 500 for female and 600 for male two days a week. That means you usually eat for five days and reduce the calories in your diet for two days.

For example, you might eat every day of the week except Tuesday and Thursday where you reduce the food you consume. You limit the calories for breakfast to 250 for women and 300 for men while dinner takes the same number of calories as well.

Eat-Stop-Eat

This method requires you to do a 24-hour fast either once or twice a week, whichever one is comfortable for you.

An example is not eating from 7 p.m. to 7 p.m. the next day. That is if you start with dinner on Monday, you don't eat from 7 p.m. Monday to 7 p.m. Tuesday. You can do this once or twice a week. If it is once, it is advisable for it to be done mid-week, like Wednesday, and if it is twice, it is good if the days are spread apart, e.g., Monday and Thursday.

You can drink water, coffee, and other noncaloric drinks between fasting periods, but solid foods are not allowed. It is, however, not advisable to start with this method as it requires a lot of energy for the long hours without food. Start with 16 hours fasting before plunging into the 24 hours fast.

Alternate-day Fasting

Most of the health benefits that were revealed are as a result of this method. That is fasting on alternate days.

There are two variations to this method;

a) 24-hour full day fasting every other day. This requires you to eat normally for a day and then fast for the next 24 hours.

b) Eating only a few hundred calories. The alternate-day fasting can be very challenging, and this made the experts devise another plan where you only eat a reduced number of calories every other day.

An example is that when you fast on Monday, you eat normally on Tuesday, fast on Wednesday, and the continue for the rest of the week.

The Warrior Diet

This method of fasting was made famous by Ori Hofmekler, another fitness expert.

This diet requires you to fast or eat a small or little chunk of food during the day while consuming a huge meal at night, a typical case of fast and feast later. You eat small amounts of fruits and vegetables during the day and fall back to a huge meal.

The meal is best eaten by 4 p.m. in the evening. No food must be eaten until the next morning when you continue with fruits and vegetables.

Feast for dinner and fast for the day.

Spontaneous Meal Skipping

This is a more natural method than the 16/8 because there's no routine. You just skip meals when convenient.

This can be done in some instances, such as when you are not really hungry or are on a journey and can't find suitable food to eat. You can skip these meals.

There's no routine to this method. You can decide to skip your meal anytime, from lunch to dinner to breakfast. Once you don't follow a routine, you are using this method.

These methods, however, are not suitable for every individual, and you don't need to try everything before you know which is ideal for you.

This guide is for women over 50 years old, and these kind of people often lose energy more rapidly than typical younger youths so methods, such as the alternate-day fasting and the eat-stop-eat method, are not suitable for women over fifty because these types and processes require a lot of energy, which these women lack.

The 16/8 is not suitable for every one woman over fifty, but it's a good start if you want to take the fast to another level. There's no magic to it, and no one can tell you what's best for you. You have to discover that yourself.

The spontaneous meal skipping is a great place to start, but the results won't be as fast as the other methods because of the lack of routine.

The best methods, however, are the eat-stop-eat and the 5:2. These two have routines you can follow, but you don't need to stay away from food, only consume small calories. This way, you fast with a routine, and the results will be achieved.

Whichever you decide to use, make sure you consult your doctor to see if intermittent fasting is suitable for you.

Chapter 07

How To Plan

Step One - Create a Monthly Calendar

On a calendar, highlight the days on which you wish to fast, depending on the type of fast you have committed yourself to. Record a start and end time on your fasting days so you know in the days leading up to your fast day what time you plan to begin and finish.

Tick off your days; this will keep you motivated and on track!

Step Two - Record Your Findings

Create a journal for your fasting journey. One or two days before the time, undertake to do your measurements. Weigh yourself first thing in the morning, after you have gone to the restroom and before breakfast. Also, do not weigh yourself wearing heavy items as they may affect the outcome of the scale.

Measure your height as this figure is related to your BMI (body mass index) result.

Record the measurements around your hips and stomach area, if you wish, you can also measure your upper thighs and arms.

Take a photo of yourself and place it into the journal too; this is not to discourage you but to keep you focused on why you began this journey.

Jot down all of these findings and update them weekly in the journal.

A journal is also the perfect way to express how you are feeling and, of course, what you are most thankful for. A journal is an important way in which to track not just the physical aspects of the diet but also the mental aspects too. Never undertake to doubt yourself; your journal should be a safe space for you to congratulate and to motivate yourself. Leave all the negative thoughts at the door!

Step Three - Plan Your Meals

The easiest way to stick to any eating program is to plan your meals; 500 calorie meals tend to be simple and easy to create but there are also many other more complex recipes for those who wish to spice things up. Who knows, perhaps you stumble across a meal you wish to eat outside of your fasting days.

It is advised that you prepare your meals the day before your fast days; doing this helps you stay committed to the fast and limits food wastage.

Initially, and in the first few weeks, it is suggested that you keep your meal preparation and recipes simple, so as not to overcomplicate the whole process. This also allows you to get used to counting your calories and knowing which foods work to keep you fuller versus those that left you feeling hungrier earlier than later.

Be sure to include your meal plan in your journal and on your calendar.

Step Four - Reward Yourself

On the days where you may return to normal eating, it is important to reward yourself. A small reward goes a long way in reminding yourself and your brain that what you are doing has merit and that it should be noticed. A reward should cater to one of our primal needs; these needs include:

- *Self-actualization*
- *Safety needs*
- *Social needs*
- *Esteem needs*

Physiological needs such as food, water, air, clothing, and shelter

Have a block of chocolate or buy yourself a new item of clothing do anything that makes your heart happy!

Step Five - Curb Hunger Pains

Initially, you will feel more discomfort when hungry, but these feelings will pass. If you do find yourself craving something, sip on black tea or coffee to help you through your day. Coffee is known to alleviate the feelings of being hungry; if you must add sweetener, do so at your discretion. Know that some sweeteners can cause the opposite effect and make you feel hungry.

Step Six - Stay Busy

Keeping busy means that the mind does not have time to dwell on your current state of affairs, especially if you find yourself reaching for a snack bar or cookie.

It is also wise to be implementing some sort of physical activity, even on your fasting days. A 20-minute walk before ending your fasting period will do wonders to help you reach the final stages of the fasting period. It can also uplift your mood when you are feeling frustrated or tense.

Step Seven - Practice Mindful Eating

As mentioned, we are inclined to eat for all sorts of reasons; happy, sad, it does not matter. The problem is that these feelings related to food become habitual, so we aren't really hungry but because we feel good or even off, we seek to tuck into something delicious.

The art of eating mindfully is to not allow these habits to master your life. The concept is simple: teach yourself to look at something, for instance, a piece of cake and think, "Do I really need it, or do I want it for other reasons?" You could decide to have a bite or two and leave the rest, but you may be less inclined to eat the whole slice (or whole cake) if you think mindfully about it.

The art of mindful eating is to revel in the food placed before you. Pay attention to colors, textures, and tastes. Savor each bite, even when eating an apple.

Your brain gradually begins to rewire itself when it comes to food and when it needs or wants something.

Practice mindful eating by:

Pay attention to where your food comes from.

Listen to what your body is telling you; stop eating when you are full.

Only eat when your body signals you to do so; when your stomach growls or if you feel faint or if your energy levels are low.

Pay attention to what is both healthy and unhealthy for us.

Consider the environmental impact our food choices make.

Every time you take a bite of your meal, set your cutlery down.

Step Eight - Practice Portion Control

Controlling portion sizes can be difficult for most; society has also regulated us to what we think is the size of an average portion should be and we have access to supersizing meals too, which does not help those struggling in the weight department. In 1961, Americans consumed 2,880 calories per day; by 2017, they were consuming 3,600 calories, which is a 34% increase and an unhealthy one at that.

To help you navigate how to better portion your food, consider trying the following: when dishing up your food, try the following trick. Half of your plate should consist of healthy fruits and/or vegetables, one quarter should be made up of your starches such as potatoes, rice, or pasta, and the remaining quarter should be made up of lean meats or seafood.

Alternatively, try the following:

Dish up onto a smaller plate or into a smaller bowl.

Say no to upsizing a meal if offered.

Buy the smaller version of the product if available or divide the servings equally into packets.

Eat half a meal at the restaurant and take the remaining half to enjoy the following day instead.

Go to bed early; it will stop any after-dinner eating.

Step Nine - Get Tech Savvy

Modern-day society has plenty to offer us in terms of the apps we can use to help determine the steps we take, the calories we burn, the calories found in our foods, as well as research, information, and motivation for lifestyle changes, especially diets and exercise. The list is endless. There are many apps on the market currently that can help you track your progress with regards to fasting.

The best intermittent fasting apps of currently (at the time of writing), and in no particular order are:

- *Zero*
- *Fast Habit*
- *Body Fast*
- *Fasting*
- *Vora*
- *Ate Food Diary*

Life Fasting Tracker

Make use of your mobile device to set reminders for yourself of when to eat, what to eat, and when your fast days are. It works especially well when using it to set reminders for when you should drink water, particularly for those who find it hard to keep their fluids up.

Making the Change

Understand that intermittent fasting is not a diet; it is a lifestyle, an eating plan that you are in control of and one that is easy to perfect. Before you know it, fasting will become second nature.

When to Start?

Begin today, not tomorrow or after a particular event or gathering. Once you have picked the fast that best suits you, begin with it immediately. Never hold off until a specific day; once you begin, you will gain momentum and it will become something that is part of your day, like many other things that fill up your day. No sweat there!

Measure Your Eating

Three days before you fast, it would be wise to begin to lessen the amount of food you are eating or dishing up less. This helps your body begin to get used to the idea that it doesn't need a whole bowl of food to get what it needs nor to feel full.

Keep up Your Exercise Plan

If you have a pre-existing exercise regime, do not alter it anyway. Simply carry on the way you were before fasting. If you are new to exercising, begin with short walks now and again, extending the time you walk. For example, take a five-minute walk, and the next day, change the time to 10 minutes of walking.

Stop, Start, Stop

Fast for a period of hours, and then eat all your calories during a certain number of hours. Consider this as a training period.

Do Your Research

Read up as much as you can about intermittent fasting this way it will put to rest any uncertainties you might have and introduce you to new ways of getting through a fasting day. Check out recipes that won't make you feel like a rabbit having to chomp on carrots all day if you are stuck with ideas of what to eat.

Have Fun

Lastly, have fun, and see what your body can do, even over 50. It is important to know that just because you are a certain age doesn't mean you are incapable of pursuing a new lifestyle change. Reward yourself when it is due, track your progress, adjust where need be, and get your beauty sleep. This is another secret to achieving overall wellness and happiness.

Know Your BMI

Your BMI is based on the measurements of your weight and height; thus, you can easily determine your body mass index, or BMI as it is more commonly known.

In total, there are four categories that an individual can fall into based on this figure. That is underweight, healthy, overweight, and obese. The concept is simple: our BMI gives us quantifiable amounts when comparing our height with our fat, muscles, bones, and organs.

How to Calculate Your BMI

To calculate your BMI, equate your weight (lbs.) x 703 divided by your height (in).

Once you have calculated your BMI, you can compare it to the body mass index chart to determine which category you are classed into.

Class	Your BMI Score
Underweight	*less than 18.5 points*
Normal weight	*18.5 – 24.9 points*

Overweight	*25 – 29.9 points*
Class 1 - Obesity	*30 – 34.9 points*
Class 2 - Obesity	*35 – 39.9 points*
Class 3 - Extreme obesity	*40+ points*

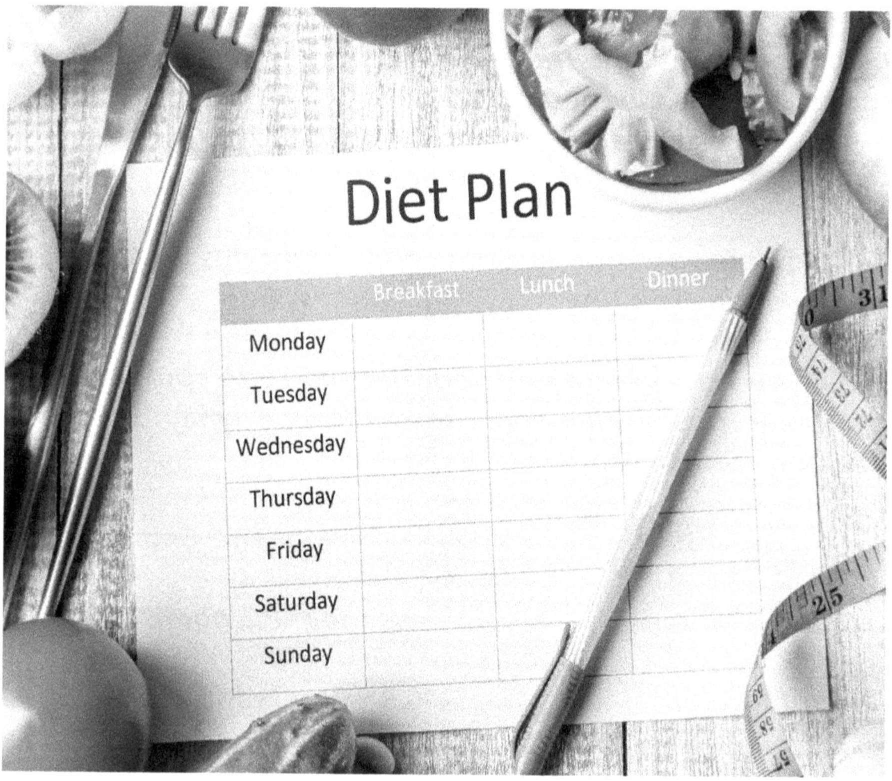

Chapter 08

Diet in Menopause

Menopause is one of the most complicated phases in a woman's life. The time when our bodies begin to change and important natural transitions occur that are too often negatively affected, while it is important to learn how to change our eating habits and eating patterns appropriately. In fact, it often happens that a woman is not ready for this new condition and experiences it with a feeling of defeat as an inevitable sign of time travel, and this feeling of prostration turns out to be too invasive and involves many aspects of one's stomach.

It is therefore important to remain calm as soon as there are messages about the first signs of change in our human body, to ward off the onset of menopause for the right purpose and to minimize the negative effects of suffering, especially in the early days. Even during this difficult transition, targeted nutrition can be very beneficial.

What Happens to The Body of a Menopausal Woman?

It must be said that a balanced diet has been carried out in life and there are no major weight fluctuations, this will no doubt be a factor supports women who are going through menopause, but that it is not a sufficient condition to present with classic symptoms that are felt, which can be classified according to the period experienced. In fact, we can distinguish between the pre-menopausal phase, which lasts around 45 to 50 years, and is physiologically compatible with a drastic reduction in the production of the hormone estrogen (responsible for the menstrual cycle, which actually starts irregularly). This period is accompanied by a series of complex and highly subjective endocrine changes. Compare effectively: headache, depression, anxiety and sleep disorders.

When someone enters actual menopause, estrogen hormone production decreases even more dramatically, the range of the symptoms widens, leading to large amounts of the hormone, for example, to a certain class called catecholamine adrenaline. The result of these changes is a dangerous heat wave, increased sweating, and the presence of tachycardia, which can be more or less severe.

However, the changes also affect the female genital organs, with the volume of the breasts, uterus and ovaries decreasing. The mucous membranes become less active and vaginal dryness increases. There may also be changes in bone balance, with decreased calcium intake and increased mobilization at the expense of the skeletal system. Because of this, there is a lack of continuous bone formation, and con-

versely, erosion begins, which is a predisposition for osteoporosis.

Although the menopause causes major changes that greatly change a woman's body and soul, metabolism is one of the worst. In fact, during menopause, the absorption and accumulation of sugars and triglycerides changes and it is easy to increase some clinical values such as cholesterol and triglycerides, which lead to high blood pressure or arteriosclerosis. In addition, many women often complain of disturbing circulatory disorders and local edema, especially in the stomach. It also makes weight gain easier, even though you haven't changed your eating habits.

The Ideal Diet for Menopause

In cases where disorders related to the arrival of menopause become difficult to manage, drug or natural therapy under medical supervision may be necessary. The contribution given by a correct diet at this time can be considerable, in fact, given the profound variables that come into play, it is necessary to modify our food routine, both in order not to be surprised by all these changes, and to adapt in the most natural way possible.

The problem of fat accumulation in the abdominal area is always caused by the drop-in estrogen. In fact, they are also responsible for the classic hourglass shape of most women, which consists in depositing fat mainly on the hips, which begins to fail with menopause. As a result, we go from a gynoid condition to an android one, with an adipose increase localized on the belly. In addition, the metabolic rate of disposal is reduced, this means that even if you do not change your diet and eat the same quantities of food as you always have, you could experience weight gain, which will be more marked in the presence of bad habits or irregular diet. The digestion is also slower and intestinal function becomes more complicated. This further contributes to swelling as well as occurrence of intolerance and digestive disorders which have never been disturbed before. Therefore, the beginning will be more problematic and difficult to manage during this period. The distribution of nutrients must be different: reducing the amount of low carbohydrate, which is always preferred not to be purified, helps avoid the peak of insulin and at the same time maintains stable blood sugar.

Furthermore, it will be necessary to slightly increase the quantity of both animal and vegetable proteins; choose good fats, preferring seeds and extra virgin olive oil and severely limit saturated fatty acids (those of animal origin such as lard, lard, etc.). All this to try to increase the proportion of antioxidants taken, which will help to counteract the effect of free radicals, whose concentration begins to increase during this period. It will be necessary to prefer foods rich in phytoestrogens, which will help to control the states of stress to which the body is subjected, and which will favor, at least in part, the overall estrogenic balance.

These molecules are divided into three main groups and the foods that contain them should never be missing on our tables: isoflavones, present mainly in legumes such as soy and red clover; lignans, of which flax seeds and oily seeds in general are particularly rich; cumestani, found in sunflower seeds, beans and sprouts. The Calcium supplementation will be necessary through cheeses such as parmesan; dairy products such as yoghurt, egg yolk, some vegetables such as rocket, Brussels sprouts, broccoli, spinach, asparagus; legumes; dried fruit such as nuts, almonds or dried grapes.

Excellent additional habits that will help to regain well-being may be: limiting sweets to sporadic occasions, thus drastically reducing sugars (for example by giving up sugar in coffee and getting used to drinking it bitterly); learn how to dose alcohol a lot (avoiding spirits, liqueurs and aperitif drinks) and choose only one glass of good wine when you are in company, this because it tends to increase visceral fat which is precisely what is going to settle at the level abdominal. Clearly, even by eating lots of fruit, it is difficult to reach a high carbohydrate quota as in a traditional diet. However, a dietary plan to follow can be useful to have a more precise indication of how to distribute the foods. Ob-

viously, one's diet must be structured in a personal way, based on specific metabolic needs and one's lifestyle.

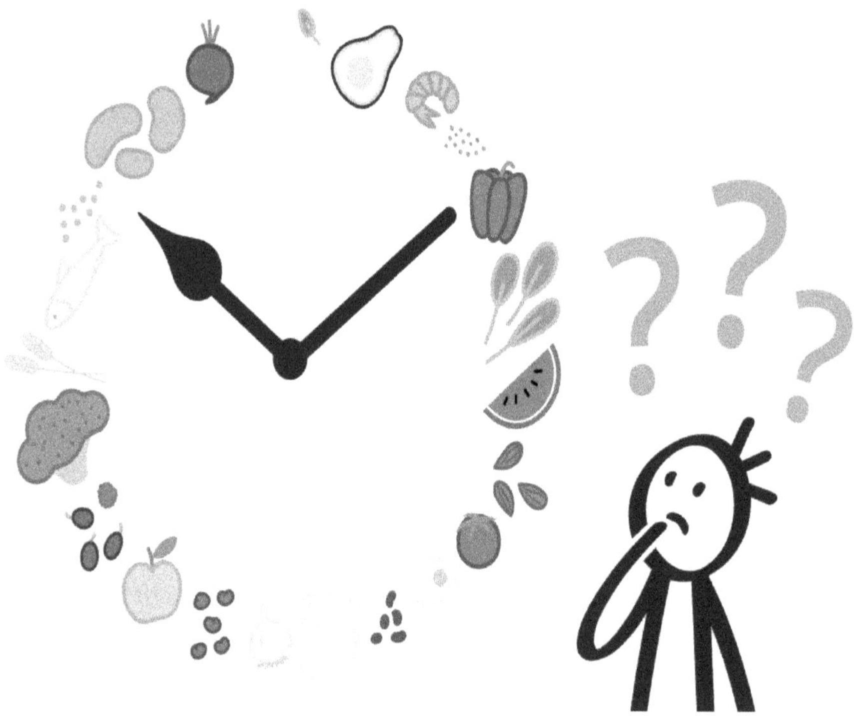

Chapter 09

Myths About Intermittent Fasting

Myth 1. Breakfast boosts metabolism

This myth is so tenacious that many people, businesses and institutions claim that breakfast is the most important meal of the day.

For example, the site of the National Nutrition Health Program strongly discourages doing without it and many manufacturers are selling their products "to start the day off on the right foot".

One can imagine that the manufacturers of breakfast cereals, margarine or spreads will not be frankly delighted if people start to skip breakfast. Rather, they have an interest in what we eat as often as possible.

By dint of hearing something, you end up believing it and you don't think about looking for evidence. But as I am stubborn, I have investigated whether the claims about breakfast are true.

In conclusion, skipping breakfast does not slow down the metabolism. It will not make you gain weight.

Myth 2. Eat 5 or 6 meals a day

According to this myth, it is necessary to eat 5 or 6 meals per day to make work the metabolism in a continuous way. This involves eating three main meals and two snacks.

Eating every few hours is believed to prevent the metabolism from slowing down. Many dietitians thus advise to eat frequently, in small portions.

There is no scientific evidence that eating 5-6 meals a day increases or maintains the speed of metabolism. In fact, the frequency of meals has no effect on metabolism.

We burn as many calories as we eat 2 or 3 times a day or we eat 5 or 6 times a day.

The only argument in favor of frequent small food intakes could be that they prevent you from being hungry (to which you can object that you are never really full because you only eat small portions).
What is proven, however, is that eating often in small portions reduces insulin sensitivity, which promotes the development of abdominal fat.

Myth 3. Eat often to avoid losing muscle mass

You may have noticed that some bodybuilders take their Tupperware with chicken breast and vegetables everywhere.

These bodybuilders want to be able to eat their protein every few hours because they fear losing muscle mass.

If you are not in the bodybuilding world, you certainly have less pressure in relation to your muscle mass. Having said that, muscle mass is important for everyone. Indeed, the amount of muscle mass you have determines your resting metabolism.

If you lose muscle mass, your resting metabolism will slow down and you will gain weight faster. Many people (not just bodybuilders) are afraid of losing muscle.

The fear of losing muscle mass is understandable. However, the fear of losing your muscles if you don't eat for a few hours has no basis.

The body stores fat for use as an energy source after digestion is complete.

It is illogical to think that if you do not eat, your body will draw on muscle mass rather than fat. This is not how the body works.

For bodybuilders, intermittent fasting has only great benefits. This is explained by the production of growth hormone. Click here to learn more about fasting and strength training.

Myth 4. When we fast, the body goes into economy mode

Prehistoric men regularly went through periods during which fasting was a necessity. For example, when you came home empty-handed from the hunt and there was nothing edible in the area.

From the point of view of evolution, our body is provided with an "energy saving mode". This mode allows the body to slow down the metabolism.

Chapter 10

Common Mistakes

Now that you know all about the process of intermittent fasting and how it should be done, you should also have the knowledge of the common mistakes that people make while doing the fast. These mistakes can actually prevent you from realizing the benefits and make the entire fast nothing but a complete waste. So, once you know what they are, make sure that you do not make the same mistakes yourself. If you do not want to make mistakes, the first and foremost thing that you need to do is be aware of everything that you are doing and also know why you are doing them. This will ensure that even if you are sometimes off the path, you can easily push yourself back on track. Also, stop beating yourself up for a cheat day or any mistake that you made. Just move on by accepting that it happened, and it cannot be undone. If you waste your energy in self-loathing, you will not be able to make plans so that the same mistake does not happen twice.

Fasting Too Long Even at the Beginning

You must have heard me saying this plenty of times already; you need to take it slow. Do not rush the process. If you haven't tried intermittent fasting ever in your life, then you should start with a 48-hour fast or even a 24-hour fast for that matter. Yes, you will have to eventually lengthen the fasting window but that does not mean you have to do it now and at once. What you have to do is increase the fasting period but do it in small increments. In case you do not follow what, I said, it will be you who will be facing certain consequences and they are bound to happen.

One of the first consequences that people have to face when they fast for longer periods too quickly is that they become grumpy. They behave badly with coworkers and loved ones. And the worst part is that you might shove it away, saying that it's just your way of coping with fasting, but it is not. Also, due to your cranky mood, some people might even give you negative feedback and in most cases, that is when people give up the fast and throw every effort down the gutter all at once. Tossing the whole idea out of the window because of such a situation is not worth it and it would not have come to it only if you had increased your fasting period gradually

The second consequence is that when people do longer fast, in the beginning, they cannot continue it after the first couple of days mainly because it becomes too unbearable for them, and they feel tremendously hungry all the time. The process of intermittent fasting should not make you feel jarred or stressed. Instead, it should be gradual and gentle.

If you truly want to continue intermittent fasting for a long stretch of time, you have to learn to make it well incorporated into your routine and for that, you need to take it slow. When you start the longer fasts right from the beginning, you are simply walking on the path of disappointment and most people give up too quickly in such cases.

Not Eating the Right Foods

This is probably the biggest mistake that I see people have been making. If you have been trying to incorporate the process of intermittent fasting into your day-to-day life, then you also have to ensure that you are eating the right foods; otherwise, it won't work the way you want it to. For starters, as you might know, fasting means that you have to learn how to get your appetite under control. And this means that you cannot simply grab that packet of chips or that bar of crunchy granola whenever you feel like. There is a time for everything, and time is highly essential. But equally essential is what you are eating in your eating window.

If you make the wrong choices, then you are definitely going to have a hard time controlling your appetite. When you are relying on foods that are rich in carbohydrates, you will be deliberately making the entire process difficult for yourself your appetite along with your levels of blood glu-

cose are in a state of continuous fluctuation. When you are on a diet that is low in carbs, you will have more fats and proteins. This will increase your levels of satiety. In simpler words, you will remain full for a longer period of time. Moreover, this will give your body flexibility in metabolism so that you can tap into your fat reserves whenever your body is fasting and does not have enough glucose as fuel.

Also, some people use intermittent fasting as an excuse to eat whatever they want when they are in the eating window. That is not right and won't bring you any good results. You have to remember that this is not a magic pill, and nothing will happen on its own if you do not put enough effort. It is true that intermittent fasting allows you to take your health into your own hands and maintain proper metabolism but for that, your diet needs to be healthy too. You have to cut down on sugar and processed foods. You need to incorporate more and more whole foods that are rich in nutrients and low in carbs.

Consuming Too Many Calories

It is important to eat the right foods so that you can get the nutrients that you need. But you should not overdo it in the eating phase. When people fast, they have this idea that they have to replenish themselves by eating an equally heavy meal in the eating window. Never try to compensate for the time you were not eating. Sometimes people end up overeating to such an extent that they not only regret their actions but also feel bloated.

Also, in case you have overeaten, don't be too harsh on yourself because it will only make matters worse. Accept the fact because you simply cannot undo it in any way. What you have to do from now on is that you have to prepare and plan your meals and keep healthy options in every meal. This will ensure that when the eating window starts, you don't have to think about what you want to eat. A very important part of the process of intermittent fasting is to figure out a balance in your routine where you can prepare healthy foods and not depend on processed foods.

Not Staying Consistent

This is probably true for everything on earth that if you are not consistent with it, it will not bring you results. The same goes for intermittent fasting. But what is worse is that if you are not consistent, then you will be stuck in a cycle where you make poor eating choices and you will be so disappointed with everything that you will not feel like doing anything about it. That is exactly something you need to avoid and for this, you have to be consistent. The best way to ensure this is to follow a fasting regime that you can maintain for the long term. You need to understand that if you truly want to reap the benefits of intermittent fasting, then it also means that you have to do it for a long period of time without giving up on it.

In case you already feel like that you will not be able to stay consistent throughout the procedure, then you need to sit down and figure out why. You need to find the reason behind it and then deal with it. Is it because you do not like the method that you have selected? If it is so, then try some other method. Or, is it because your fasting and feeding window is wrong and you are having a hard time adjusting to it? In that case, you need to adjust the timings in a different manner. Whatever it is, just don't give up before figuring out the why.

Doing Too Many Things at the Same Time

This is also one of the reasons why people give up on intermittent fasting, especially beginners. There is a saying that you should not bite off more than you can chew, and this is exactly what I am talking about here. If you are trying out intermittent fasting for the first time and you are also trying to maintain a daily gym schedule (which you don't usually do) and on top that, you are also trying to cook your own meals (when you are habituated to take-outs), then it is very easy to feel stressed.

So, maybe you can start by training only three times a week and then you can take the help of your family members in cooking your meals. If you do not have anyone living with you, then you can skip the gym for now and maybe go for a run in the neighborhood in the initial days. Once you are okay with this routine, then you can incorporate the gym.

Now that you know the common mistakes, I hope this will help you to avoid.

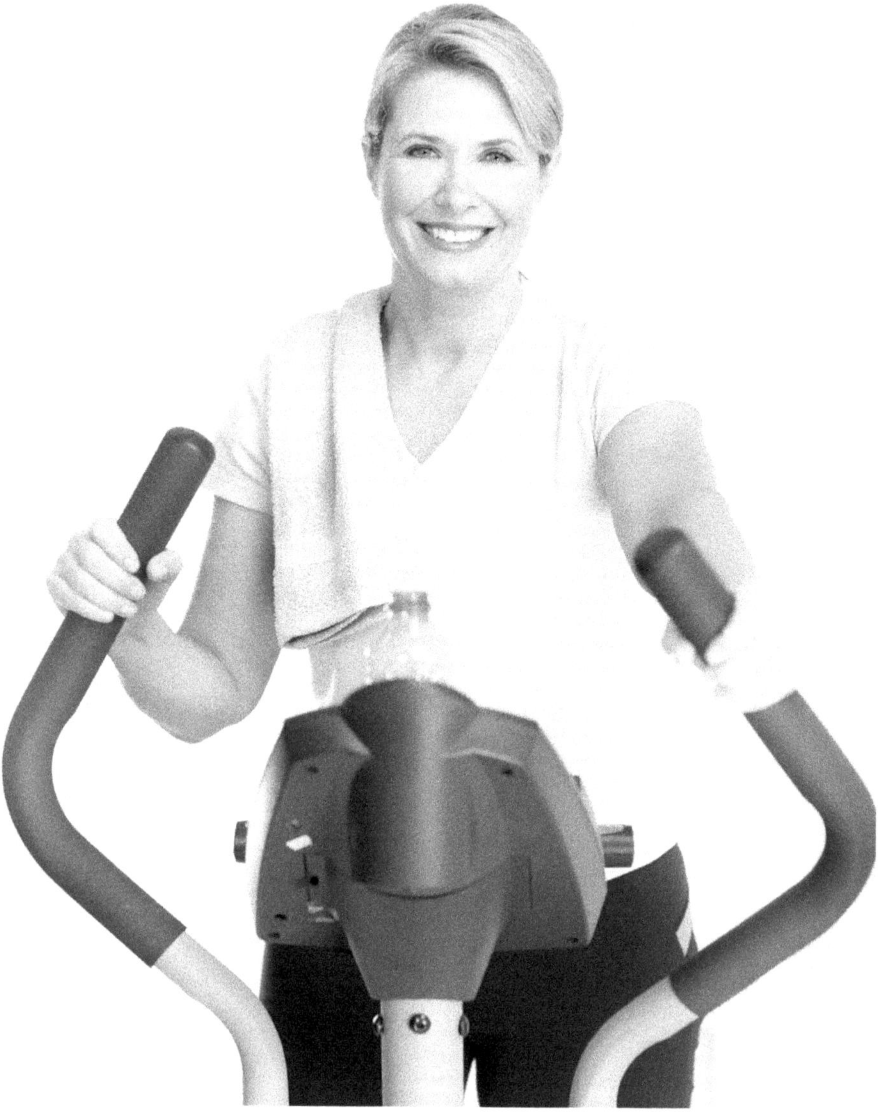

Chapter 11

Intermittent Fasting and Exercise

Many people will ask if it is safe to combine fasting with exercise. I am here to say it is. Yet, some factors need to be considered before combining the two. First, the type of fasting regimen should be considered alongside the physical, mental, and psychological health of the individual. Women with existing medical conditions should not combine fasting with exercises before being advised by a medical expert. So, while it is safe to practice intermittent fasting and include exercise if you are an already active person, doing so is not suitable for everyone.

First of all, your metabolism can be negatively impacted if you exercise and fast for long periods. For example, if you exercise daily while fasting for more than a month, your metabolic rate can begin to slow down.

Combining the two can trigger a higher rate of breaking down glycogen and body fat. This means that you burn fat at an accelerated rate. Also, when you combine these two, your growth hormones are boosted. This results in improved bone density. Your muscles are also positively impacted when you exercise. Your muscles will become more resilient to stress and age slower. This is also a quick way to trigger autophagy keeping brain cells and tissues strong, making you feel, and look younger.

Exercise is Even Better After 50

Cardiovascular exercise is best for the heart and lungs. It improves oxygen delivery to specific parts of your body, reduces stress, improves sleep, burns fat, and improves sex drive. Some of the more common cardio exercises are running, brisk walking, and swimming. In the gym, machines such as the elliptical, treadmill, and Stairmaster are used to help with cardio. Some people are satisfied and feel like they've done enough after 20 minutes on the treadmill, but if you want to continue to be strong and independent as you grow older, you need to consider adding strength training to your workout. After 50, strength training for a woman is no longer about six-pack abs, building biceps, or vanity muscles. Instead, it has switched to maintaining a body that is healthy, strong, and is less prone to injury and illness.

Women over 50 who engage in strength training for 20 to 30 minutes a day can reap the following benefits:

1. *Reduced body fat: Accumulating excess body fat is not healthy for any woman at any age. To prevent many of the diseases associated with aging, it is important to maintain a healthy body weight by burning excess fat.*
2. *Build bone density: With stronger bones, accidental*

falls are less likely to result in broken limbs or a visit to the emergency room.

3. *Build muscle mass : Although you are not likely to be the next champion bodybuilder, strength training will make you an overall stronger woman who will carry herself with ease, push your lawnmower, lift your groceries, and perform all other tasks that require you to exert some strength.*
4. *Significant less risk of chronic diseases: In addition to keeping chronic diseases away, strength training can also reduce symptoms of some diseases you may have, such as back pain, obesity, arthritis, osteoporosis, and diabetes. Of course, the type of exercises you do if you have any chronic disease should be recommended by your doctor.*
5. *Boosts mental health: A loss of self-confidence and depression are some psychological issues that come along with aging. Women who keep themselves fit with exercises tend to be generally more self-assured and are less likely to develop depression.*

Strength Training Exercises for Women Over 50

These ten strength training exercises you can do right in the comfort of your home. All you need is a mat, a chair, and some hand weights of about 3 – 8 pounds. As you get stronger, you can increase the weight. Take a minute to rest before switching between each routine. Ensure that you move slowly through the exercises, breathe properly, and focus on maintaining the right form. If you start to feel lightheaded or dizzy during your routines, especially if you are performing the exercise during your fasting window, discontinue immediately.

Squat to Chair

This exercise is great for improving your bone health. A lot of age-related bone fractures and falls in women involve the pelvis, so this exercise will target and strengthen your pelvic bone and the surrounding muscles.

To perform this:

1. *Stand fully upright in front of a chair as if you are ready to sit and spread your feet shoulder-width apart.*
2. *Extend your arms in front of you and keep them that way all through the movement.*
3. *Bend your knees and slowly lower your hips as if you want to sit on the chair, but don't sit. When your butt touches the chair slightly, press into your heels to get back your initial standing position. Repeat that for about 10 to 15 times.*

Forearm Plank

This exercise targets your core and shoulders.

Here's how to do it:

1. *Get into a push-up position, but with your arms bent at the elbows such that your forearm is supporting your weight.*
2. *Keep your body off the mat or floor and keep your back straight at all times. Don't raise or drop your hips. This will engage your core. Hold the position for 30 seconds and then drop to your knees. Repeat ten times.*

Modified Push-ups

This routine targets your arms, shoulders, and core.

How's how to do it:

1. *Kneel on your mat. Place your hands on the mat below your shoulders and let your knees be behind your hips so that your back is stretched at an angle.*
2. *Tuck your toes under and tighten your abdominal muscles. Gradually bend your elbows as you lower your chest toward the floor.*
3. *Push back on your arms to press your chest back to your previous position. Repeat for as many times as is comfortable.*

Bird Dog

When done correctly, this exercise can strengthen the muscles of your posterior chain as it targets your back and core. It may seem easy at first but can be a bit tricky.

To do this correctly:

1. *Go on all fours on your mat.*
2. *Tighten your abdominal muscles and shift your weight to your right knee and left hand. Slowly extend your right hand in front of you and your left leg behind you. Ensure that both your hands and legs are extended as far as possible and stay in that position for about 5 seconds. Return to your starting position. This is one repetition. Switch to your left knee and right hand and repeat the movement. Alternate between both sides for 20 repetitions.*

Shoulder Overhead Press

This targets your biceps, shoulders, and back.

To perform this move:

1. *With dumbbells in both hands, stand and spread your feet shoulder-width apart.*
2. *Bring the dumbbells up to the sides of your head and tighten your abdominal muscles.*

3. *Slowly press the dumbbells up until your arms are straight above your head. Slowly return to the first position. Repeat 10 times. You can also do this exercise while sitting.*

Chest Fly

This targets your chest, back, core, and glutes.

To do this:

1. *Lie with your back flat on your mat, your knees at an angle close to 90 degrees, and your feet firmly planted on the floor or mat.*
2. *Hold dumbbells in both hands over your chest. Keep your palms facing each other and gently open your hands away from your chest. Let your upper arms touch the floor without releasing the tension in them.*
3. *Contract your chest muscles and slowly return the dumbbells to the initial position. Repeat for about ten times.*

Standing Calf Raise

This exercise improves the mobility of your lower legs and feet and also improves your stability.

Here's how to perform it.

1. *Hold a dumbbell in your left hand and place your right hand on something sturdy to give you balance.*
2. *When you are sure of your balance, lift your left foot off the floor with the dumbbell hanging at your side. Stand erect and move your weight such that you are almost standing on your toes.*
3. *Slowly return to the starting position. Do this 15 times before switching to the other leg and doing the same thing all over again.*

Single-Leg Hamstring Bridge

This move targets your glutes, quads, and hamstrings.

To do this:

1. *Lie flat on your back. Place your feet flat on the floor or mat and spread your bent knees apart.*
2. *Place your arms flat by your side and lift one leg straight.*
3. *Contract your glutes as you lift your hips into a bridge position with your arms still in position. Hold for about 2 to 3 seconds and drop your hips to the mat. Repeat about ten times before switching your leg. Do the same again.*

Bent-Over Row

This targets your back muscles and spine.

To do this:

1. *Hold dumbbells in both hands and stand behind a sturdy object (for example, a chair). Bend forward and rest your head on the chosen object. Relax your neck and slightly bend your knees. With both palms facing each other pull the dumbbells to touch your ribs. Hold the position for about 2 to 5 seconds and slowly return to the starting position. Repeat 10 to 15 times.*

Basic Ab

A distended belly is a common occurrence in older women. This exercise can strengthen and tighten the abdominal muscles bringing them inward toward your spine.

To perform this:

1. *Lie on your back with your feet firmly planted on the floor and your knees bent. Relax your upper body and rest your hands on your thighs.*
2. *As you exhale, lift yourself upward off the mat or floor. Stop the upward movement when your hands are resting on your knees. Hold the position for about 2 to 5 seconds and then slowly return to the starting position. Repeat for about 20 to 30 times.*

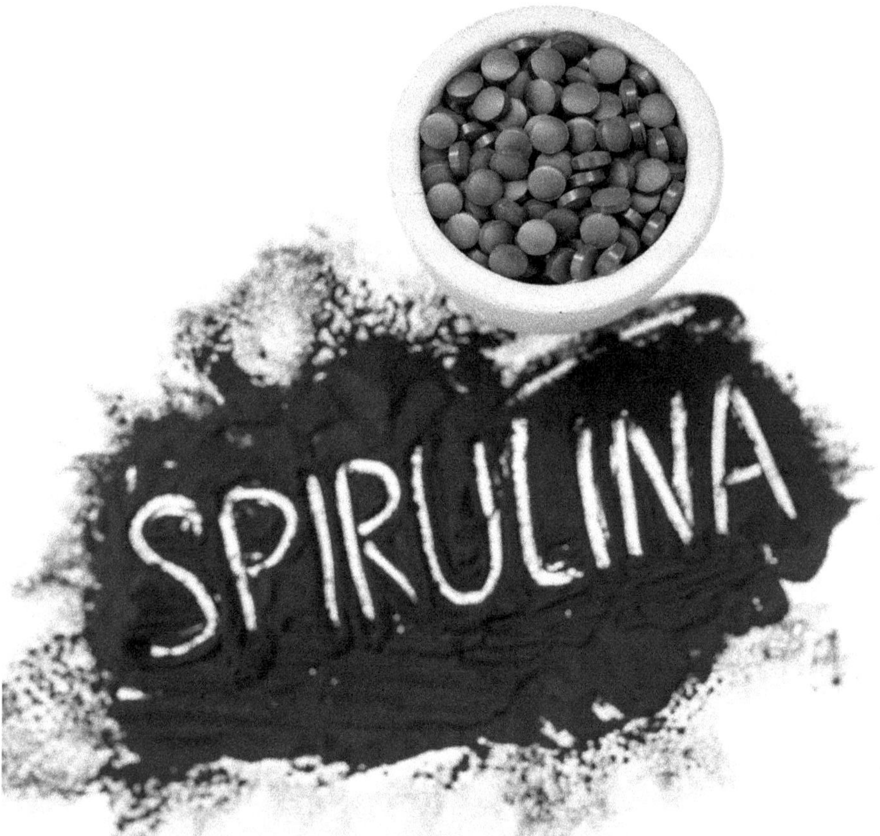
SPIRULINA

Chapter 12

Spirulina Algae. The Supplement That Helps You Fast

Spirulina (pronounced spear-uh-lee-nun) is an edible type of cyanobacteria, a single-celled, blue-green microalgae that is found naturally in both in salt and fresh waters. This spiral-shaped microalgae are cultivated and harvested throughout the world as both a supplement and a whole food. Because it has a soft cell wall made of protein and complex sugars, it can be digested efficiently. It is widely considered a green superfood with positive health benefits because of its richness in:

- *Protein (dried spirulina contains between 50% to 70% protein)*
- *Minerals (especially Iron and Manganese)*
- *Vitamins (especially Vitamins B1, and B2)*
- *Carotenoids*
- *Antioxidants*

Spirulina is used internationally in nutrition drinks, pasta, crackers, noodles, nutrition bars, broths, cakes, pet foods, and cereal. It is also used as a component in food coloring, cosmetics, skin creams, shampoos, personal care products, and more. Spirulina can be purchased at most specialty nutrition stores, some supermarket chains, as well as on-line. It is typically sold in powder or tablet form.

As a food, eating spirulina is nothing new. Historians indicate that spirulina was part of the diet of the Kamen Empire of Chad in the ninth century (AD/CE). In 1519, Hernando Cortez and his Spanish Conquistadors observed that spirulina was eaten by Aztecs around Lake Texcoco, which is modern day Mexico City. Today, more than one thousand metric tons of spirulina are harvested worldwide in natural lakes, commercial farms, village farms, and family microforms.

Spirulina farming is much more environmentally friendly compared to conventional food production. Most conventional foods are generated using chemicals including pesticides, antibiotics, preservatives, additives, and fungicides. Not only have these chemicals been shown to have negative impacts on health, but they also cause damage to our water supply and the overall natural environment. Harvesting spirulina offers more nutrition per acre, and doesn't incur environmental costs associated with toxic cleanup, water treatment, or subsidies, that other food industries require.

The growing popularity of spirulina as a green superfood has taken off over the past forty years. Scientific research conducted in recent decades supports the many health benefits of spirulina, adding to its growing use as a food or supplement. Research is ongoing, and in some cases, has not been tested on human subjects. Additionally, the U.S. FDA has not approved spirulina as a medicine or treatment for diseases (although it is an approved supplement and food). However, the health benefits that research has uncovered so far have been very positive, showing some transformative results.

Cancer Fighter

Spirulina is high in beta-carotene, a type of phytochemical, that is believed to help protect the body against free radicals that can come from various forms of pollution including cigarette smoke and herbicides. Spirulina's effects on cancer has been demonstrated in animals and humans with positive effects indicating reduction in cancer cells, and even in some cases, reversal of oral cancer.

Diabetes and Blood Sugar Improvement

A study from the University of Baroda in India revealed that spirulina may help diabetics. Over the course of a two-month study, patients with type 2 diabetes who were given two grams of spirulina every day improved blood sugar and lipid levels.

Immune System Boost

Tests on animals and senior citizens have exhibited a boost of immune system, which is crucial to preventing viral infections. In these studies, spirulina was shown to increase the production of antibodies, which are needed to fight viral and bacterial infections, as well as some chronic illnesses.

Anti-Virus

Not only has the algae been observed to boos antibodies, but it has also shown an ability to hinder the replication of viruses. The National Cancer Institute (NCI) publicized that spirulina was "remarkably active" against the AIDS virus (HIV-1) after conducting a study in 1989. Test tube experiments have also shown spirulina to inhibit the replication of other viruses including influenza A, mumps, and measles.

Antihistamine

In several scientific studies, spirulina appeared to help allergy symptoms such as watery eyes, skin reactions, and runny nose. In a recent study, a group of people suffering from rhinitis, an inflammation of the nasal mucous membrane, saw significant improvements of their allergy symptoms when given a daily 1000 mg or 2000 mg doses of spirulina over the course of twelve weeks.

Blood Pressure Reduction

Participants in an experiment at the National Autonomous University of Mexico were able to drop their blood pressure after taking spirulina for six weeks, without any other changes in their diet. Spirulina increases the body's production of nitric oxide, which is a gas that can widen blood vessels. Widened blood vessels improve the body's flow of blood, and ultimately can reduce blood pressure.

Lower Cholesterol

Recent research conducted in Greek universities has shown some promising effects on adults with high cholesterol. Over the course of three months, fifty-two adults were given one gram of spirulina each day. At the end of the three-month study period, the group's average triglycerides decreased over 16% and low-density lipoprotein (LDL) cholesterol (also known as the "bad" cholesterol) by 10%.

Radiation Treatment

After the Russian Chernobyl nuclear disaster in 1986, the Russian government turned to spirulina to treat children who had been exposed to the radiation. Radiation destroys bone marrow, thus complicating the body's ability to create normal white or red blood cells. Within six weeks, children who were fed five grams of spirulina every day were able to make remarkable recoveries. The blue pigment of spirulina is comprised of phycocyanin, which enables the body to cleanse some radioactive metals.

Kidney and Liver Detoxification

Not only has spirulina's phycocyanin been shown to cleanse radioactive metals, it may also have the ability to cleanse heavy metal poisoning. Studies in Japan and elsewhere suggest that spirulina is able to safely assist in the removal of heavy metals such as arsenic, lead, mercury and other similar metals that can be found in medicine, dental fillings, fish, deodorants, cigarettes, and drinking water.

Reducing Malnutrition

According to the United Nations Food and Agricultural Organization, over 800 million people worldwide suffer from chronic undernourishment. Malnutrition is an epidemic as millions of people around the world lack enough proteins and micronutrients such as vitamins and minerals. With spirulina containing a significant amount of protein, B-vitamins, and iron, one tablespoon a day could eliminate micronutrient deficiencies that cause diseases such as anemia. Unlike other protein foods such as beef or nuts, spirulina is a very digestible source of protein. The digestive tract of malnourished individuals exhibits malabsorption, making the easily digestible spirulina, an even more attractive source of nourishment.

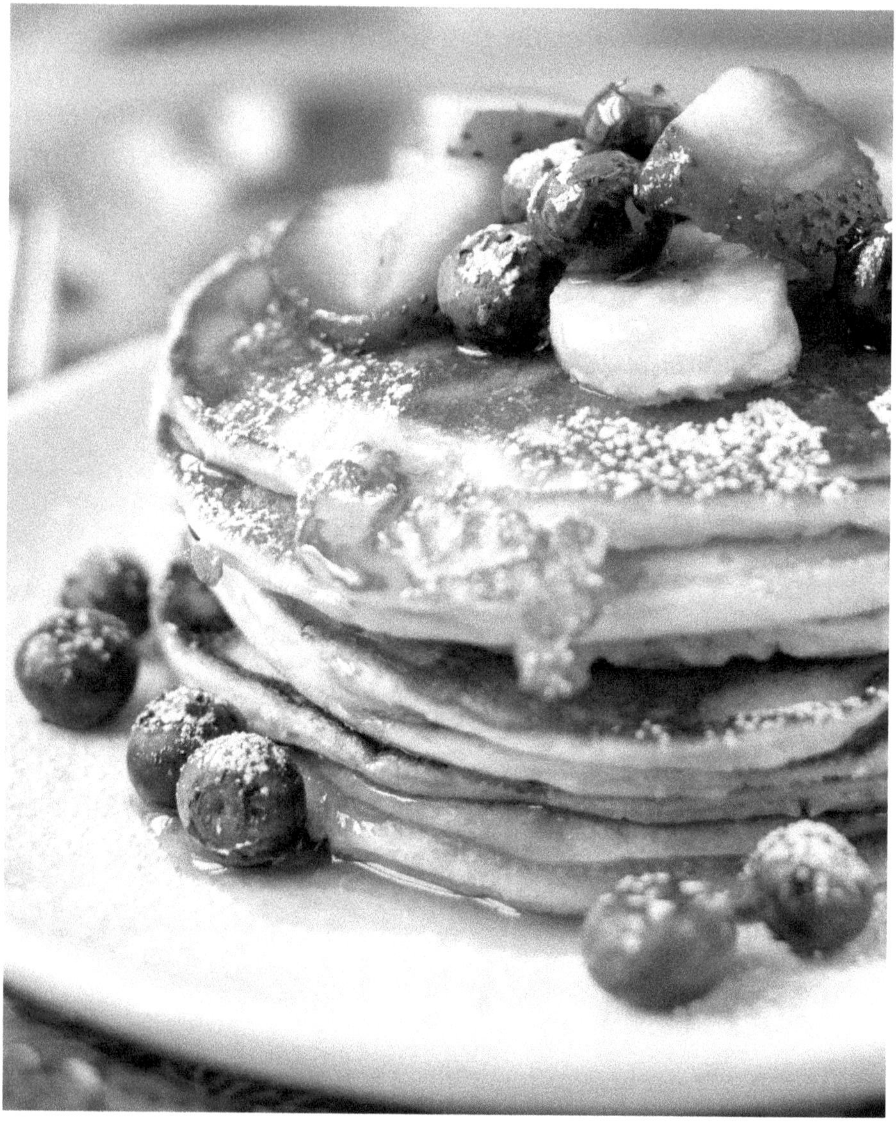

Chapter 13

Breakfast Recipes

1.Pancakes

Preparation time: *5 minutes*
Cooking time: *15 minutes*
Servings: *4*
Ingredients:

- *Egg – 1 large*
- *Egg whites – 2*
- *Cream cheese – 2 tbsp*
- *Unsweetened, canned pumpkin – 3 tbsp (not pie filling)*
- *Vanilla extract – 1 tbsp*
- *Almond flour - 2/3 cup*
- *Coconut flour – 2 tbsp*
- *Swerve sweetener – 1 tbsp*
- *Pumpkin pie spice – 1 tsp*
- *Salt – 1/8 tsp*
- *Baking powder – 1 tsp*
- *Baking soda – ¼ tsp*
- *Xanthan gum – ½ tsp*
- *Water as needed*

Topping:

- *Cream cheese – 1/3 cup*
- *Unsweetened canned pumpkin – 2 tbsp*
- *Swerve sweetener – 1 to 1 ½ tbsp*
- *Cinnamon – ½ tsp*
- *Pumpkin pie spice – 1/8 tsp*
- *Vanilla extract – ½ tsp*

Directions:

Preheat a griddle to 350°F and spray with non-stick cooking spray.

Add all the wet pancake ingredients except water into a blender and blend. Then add the dry ingredients and blend until smooth.

Add water a little at a time until the pancake batter has the right consistency.

Pour a small amount of batter onto heated griddle.

Cook until browned and the edges (almost to the center) are dry about 3 to 4 minutes.

Then flip and cook for 2 to 3 minutes more.

For the topping: in a processor, add all topping ingredients and blend until creamy.

Top the pancakes with toppings and drizzle with maple syrup.

Nutrition:
Calories 206 Total Fat 14.4g Saturated Fat 7.5g Cholesterol 73mg Sodium 289mg Total Carbohydrate 11.1g Dietary Fiber 4.4g Total Sugars 1.4g Protein 7.6g

2.Oatmeal

Preparation time: *5 minutes*
Cooking time: *10 minutes*
Servings: *6*
Ingredients:

- *Chia seeds - 1/3 cup*
- *Crushed pecans - 1 cup*
- *Cauliflower - 1/2 cup, riced*
- *Flaxseed meal - 1/3 cup*
- *Coconut milk - 3 1/2 cups*
- *Butter - 3 tbsp*
- *Heavy cream - 1/4 cup*
- *Cream cheese - 3 oz.*
- *Maple flavor - 1 tsp*
- *Cinnamon - 1 1/2 tsp*
- *Erythritol - 3 tbsp powdered*
- *Vanilla - 1/2 tsp*
- *Allspice - 1/4 tsp*
- *Nutmeg - 1/4 tsp*
- *Liquid stevia - 10-15 drops*
- *Xanthan gum - 1/8 tsp (optional)*

Directions:

In a medium saucepan, heat milk over medium heat.

Crush pecans and add to the pan. Lower heat to toast.

Now add cauliflower to the coconut milk and bring to a boil. Reduce to simmer, add spices and mix.

Grind erythritol and add to the pan. Then add chia seeds, flax, stevia and mix well.

Add butter, cream, and cream cheese to the pan and mix well.

Add xanthan gum to make it a bit thicker.

Serve.

Nutrition:
Calories 485 Total Fat 46.5g Saturated Fat 22.5g Cholesterol 38mg Sodium 174mg Total Carbohydrate 21.7g Dietary Fiber 9.4g Total Sugars 10.7g Protein 7.7g

3. Veggie Omelet

Preparation time: *5 minutes*
Cooking time: *12 minutes*
Servings: *1*
Ingredients

- *Eggs – 3*
- *Almond milk or water – 1 tbsp*
- *Kosher salt – ½ tsp*
- *Freshly ground black pepper – ½ tsp*
- *Unsalted butter – 3 tbsp*
- *Swiss chard – 1 bunch, cleaned and stemmed*
- *Ricotta – 1/3 cup*

Directions:

Crack the eggs in a bowl. Add water or milk, season with salt and pepper. Beat with a fork and set aside.

Melt 2 tbsp butter over medium-high heat in an 8-inch non-stick skillet.

Add a few of the swiss chard and continue to sauté until just wilted. Remove from pan. Set aside.

Melt 1 tbsp butter in the skillet.

Then slowly add the egg mixture and tilt the pan, so the mixture spreads evenly. Allow the egg to firm up a bit. Cook for another 1 minute.

Spoon in the ricotta when the edges are firm, but the center is still a bit runny.

With a spatula, fold about 1/3 of the omelet over the ricotta filling.

Serve on a plate with Swiss chard.

Nutrition:
Calories 652 Total Fat 57.9g Saturated Fat 33.2g Cholesterol 608mg Sodium 1776mg Total Carbohydrate 8.2g Dietary Fiber 1.2g Total Sugars 2.2g Protein 27.5g

4.Ham Omelet

Preparation time: *5 minutes*
Cooking time: *10 minutes*
Servings: *5*
Ingredients:

- *Unsalted butter – 1 ½ tbsp*
- *Eggs – 10*
- *Milk – 2 tbsp*
- *Kosher salt – 1 tsp*
- *Freshly ground black pepper – ¼ tsp*
- *Cooked ham – 1 ¼ cups, diced*
- *Shredded sharp cheddar – 1 ½ cups*
- *Fresh chives – 1/3 cup, chopped*

Directions:
Melt the butter in a skillet. Add ham and sauté until browned.

Meanwhile, whisk together the eggs, pepper, kosher salt, and milk in a bowl.

Pour into the pan and cook for 4 to 5 minutes, or until the desired doneness. Stirring occasionally.

Just before the eggs are set, add chives and cheddar.
Nutrition: *Calories 175 Total Fat 9.4g Saturated Fat 5.1g Cholesterol 38mg Sodium 1084mg Total Carbohydrate 3.1g Dietary Fiber 0.6g Total Sugars 1g Protein 19g*

5.Low-Carb Cheese & Bacon Stuffed Meat Pies

Preparation Time: *10 mins*
Cooking Time: *40 min*
Servings: *4*
Ingredient:

Filling:

- *500 g ground beef (1.1 lb.)*
- *4 large slices bacon, chopped (120 g/ 4.2 oz.)*
- *1 mall brown onion, chopped (g/ oz.)*
- *1 tbsp coconut amines (15 ml)*
- *2 tbsp tomato sauce/passata (30 ml)*
- *1 cup beef stock or ban broth (240 ml/ 8 Fl oz)*
- *½ tsp xanthan gum*

Pie crust:

- *2 ¼ cups shredded mozzarella cheese (250g/8.8oz)*
- *1 cup 2 tbsp shredded edam cheese (125g/4.4oz)*
- *1/3 cup 1 tbsp full-fat cream cheese (100g/3.5oz)*
- *1 ½ cups almond flour (150g/5.3oz)*
- *2 large eggs*
- *1 tsp onion powder*
- *6 small chunks of sharp cheddar (66g/2.3oz)*

Directions:

Cut the bacon into small strips and dice the onion.

Add to a skillet, along with the ground beef. Cook until just browned.

Add coconut aminos, passata, beef stock, and xanthan gum and stir well to combine. Bring to boil then reduce the heat and simmer for 30 minutes.

Remove from the heat and let cool. Once mixture is cool, heat oven to 200 °C/ 390 °F (fan assisted).

Prepare the pie crust. Place the cheeses and cream cheese into a large bowl and microwave for 1 minute. Remove and stir, then return for another 30 seconds. Repeat this once more. Add the almond meal, onion powder and eggs and mix well until you have a soft dough.

Divide into four parts and sit one portion aside. Cut each of the remaining three portions in half and then flatten them out into large circles (you will have a total of six circles).

Spray a six-hole oversized muffin pan and press the dough into each cup, making sure to leave overhang at the top as the dough will shrink while cooking. Bake for 10 minutes.

Remove and spoon some filling into each cup. Press a chunk of cheddar into the centre.

Then top with the remaining filling.

Divide the reserved dough into six and flatten out into lids.

Lay the lid on top of the pies and gently press around the edges to seal. Cut a couple of steam vents in top of each pie.

Return to the oven for 10-15 minutes until golden brown on top.

Eat warm, with sugar-free ketchup if you want to feel very Australian. If you can't find sugar-free, you can make your own keto ketchup in just a few minutes!

Store in the refrigerator for up to 5 days.

Nutrition:
Net carbs: 2.3g Protein: 9.9g Fat: 8.2g Calories: 123kcal

6.Avocado Egg Bowls

Preparation time: *5 minutes*
Cooking time: *10 minutes*
Servings: *3*
Ingredients:

- *1 tsp coconut oil*
- *2 organics, free-range*
- *Salt and pepper*
- *1 Large & ripe avocado*
- *For Garnishing:*
- *Chopped walnuts*
- *Balsamic Pearls*
- *Fresh thyme*

Directions:
Slice your avocado in two, then take out the pit and remove enough of the inside so that there is enough space inside to accommodate an entire egg.

Cut off a little bit of the bottom of the avocado so that the avocado will sit upright as you place it on a stable surface.

Open your eggs and put each of the yolks in a separate bowl or container. Place the egg whites in the same small bowl. Sprinkle some pepper and salt to the whites, according to your personal taste, then mix them well.

Melt the coconut oil in a pan that has a lid that fits and put it on med-high.

Put in the avocado boats, with the meaty side down on the pan, the skin side up and sauté them for approx. 35 seconds, or when they become darker in color.

Turn them over, then add to the spaces inside, almost filling the inside with the whites of the eggs.

Then, reduce the temperature and place the lid. Let them sit covered it for approx. 16 to 20 minutes until the whites are just about fully cooked.

Gently add one yolk onto each of the avocados and keep cooking them for 4 to 5 mins, just until they get to the point of cook you want them at.

Move the avocados to a dish and add toppings to each of them using the walnuts, the balsamic pearls, or/and thyme.

Nutrition:
Calories 215 Fat 18g Carbohydrates 8g Protein 9g

7.Chia Seed Banana Blueberry Delight

Preparation Time: *30 minutes*
Cooking Time:
Servings: *2*
Ingredients:

- *1 cup yogurt*
- *½ cup blueberries*
- *1/2 tsp Salt*
- *1/2 tsp Cinnamon*
- *1 banana*
- *1 tsp Vanilla Extract*
- *1/4 cup Chia Seeds*

Directions:
Discard the skin of the banana.

Cut into semi thick circles.

You can mash them or keep them as whole if you like to bite into your fruits.

Clean the blueberries properly and rinse well.

Soak the chia seeds in water for 30 minutes or longer.

Drain the chia seeds and transfer into a bowl.

Add the yogurt and mix well.

Add the salt, cinnamon and vanilla and mix again.

Now fold in the bananas and blueberries gently.

If you want add dried fruit or nuts, add it and then serve immediately.

This is best served cold.

Nutrition:
Calories 260 Fats 26.6g Carbohydrates 17.4g Protein 4.1g

8.Savory Breakfast Muffins

Preparation time: *10 minutes*
Cooking time: *35 minutes*
Servings: *6*
Ingredients:

- *8 eggs*
- *1 cup shredded cheese*
- *Salt and pepper to taste*
- *½ tsp baking powder*
- *¼ cup diced onion*
- *2/3 cup coconut flour*
- *1 ½ cup spinach*
- *¼ cup full fat coconut milk*
- *1 tbsp basil, chopped*
- *½ cup cooked chicken, diced finely*

Directions:
Preheat the oven to 375-degree F.

Use butter or oil to grease your muffin tray or you can use muffin paper liners.

In a large mixing bowl, whisk the eggs.

Add in the coconut milk and mix again.
Gradually shift in the coconut flour with baking powder salt.

Add in the cooked chicken, onion, spinach, basil and combine well.

Add the cheese and mix again.

Pour the mixture onto your muffin liners.

Bake for about 25 minutes.

Serve at room temperature.

Nutrition:
Calories 388 Fat 25.8g Carbohydrate 8.6g Proteins 25.3g

9.Morning Meatloaf

Preparation Time: *10 minutes*
Cooking Time: *20 minutes*
Servings: *6*
Ingredients:

- *1 ½ pound of breakfast sausage*
- *6 large organic eggs*
- *2 tablespoons of unsweetened non-dairy milk*
- *1 small onion, finely chopped*
- *2 medium garlic cloves, peeled and minced*
- *4-ounces of cream cheese, softened and cubed*
- *1 cup of shredded cheddar cheese*
- *2 tablespoons of scallions, chopped*
- *1 cup of water*

Directions:

Add all the ingredients apart from water in a large bowl. Stir until well combined.

Form the sausage mixture into a meatloaf and wrap with a sheet of aluminum foil. Ensure that the meatloaf fits inside your Instant Pot. If not, remove parts of the mixture and reserve for future use.

Once you wrap the meatloaf into a packet, add 1 cup of water and a trivet to your Instant Pot. Put the meatloaf on the trivet's top.

Cover and cook for 25 minutes on high pressure. When done, quick release the pressure. Carefully remove the lid.

Unwrap the meatloaf and check if the meatloaf is done. Serve and enjoy!

Nutrition:
Calories 592 Carbohydrates 2.5g Proteins 11g Fats 49.5g

10.Green Pineapple

Preparation Time: *5 minutes*
Cooking Time: *0 minutes*
Servings: *3*
Ingredients:

- *1/2 of a pineapple*
- *1 broccoli, diced*
- *1 cup water*
- *1 long cucumber, diced*
- *A dash of salt*
- *1 kiwi, diced*

Directions:
Add kiwi, cucumber, pineapple, broccoli and water in a blender.

Add the salt and blend until smooth.

Serve.

Nutrition:
Calories 251 Fats 0.4g Proteins 0.5g Carbohydrates 22g

Chapter 14

Lunch Recipes

11.Salmon with Sauce

Preparation time: *5 minutes*
Cooking time: *15 minutes*
Servings: *2*
Ingredients:

- *Salmon fillet - 1 1/2 lb.*
- *Duck fat - 1 tbsp*
- *Dried dill weed - ¾ to 1 tsp*
- *Dried tarragon - ¾ to 1 tsp*
- *Salt and pepper to taste*
- *Cream Sauce:*
- *Heavy cream - 1/4 cup*
- *Butter - 2 tbsp*
- *Dried dill weed - 1/2 tsp*
- *Dried tarragon - 1/2 tsp*
- *Salt and pepper to taste*

Directions:
Slice the salmon in half and make 2 fillets. Season skin side with salt and pepper and meat of the fish with spices.

In a skillet, heat 1 tbsp duck fat over medium heat.

Add salmon to the hot pan, skin side down.

Cook the salmon for about 5 minutes. When the skin is crisp, lower the heat and flip salmon. Cook salmon on low heat for 7 to 15 minutes or until your desired doneness is reached.

Remove salmon from the pan and set aside.

Add spices and butter to the pan and let brown. Once browned, add cream and mix.

Top salmon with sauce and serve.

Nutrition:
Calories 449 Total Fat 34.5g Saturated Fat 14.4g Cholesterol 136mg Sodium 168mg Total Carbohydrate 1.1g Dietary Fiber 0.1g Total Sugars 0g Protein 35.2g

12.Butter Chicken

Preparation time: *5 minutes*
Cooking time: *30 minutes*
Servings: *4*
Ingredients:

- *Butter – ¼ cup*
- *Mushrooms – 2 cups, sliced*
- *Chicken thighs – 4 large*
- *Onion powder – ½ tsp*
- *Garlic powder – ½ tsp*
- *Kosher salt – 1 tsp*
- *Black pepper – ¼ tsp*
- *Water – ½ cup*
- *Dijon mustard – 1 tsp*
- *Fresh tarragon – 1 tbsp, chopped*

Directions:
Season the chicken thighs with onion powder, garlic powder, salt, and pepper.

In a sauté pan, melt 1 tbsp butter.

Sear the chicken thighs about 3 to 4 minutes per side, or until both sides are golden brown. Remove the thighs from the pan.

Add the remaining 3 tbsp of butter to the pan and melt.

Add the mushrooms and cook for 4 to 5 minutes or until golden brown. Stirring as little as possible.

Add the Dijon mustard and water to the pan. Stir to deglaze.

Place the chicken thighs back in the pan with the skin side up.

Cover and simmer for 15 minutes.

Stir in the fresh herbs. Let sit for 5 minutes and serve.

Nutrition:
Calories 414 Total Fat 32.9g Saturated Fat 13.6g Cholesterol 149mg Sodium 786mg Total Carbohydrate 2g Dietary Fiber 0.5g Total Sugars 0.8g Protein 26.5g

13.Lamb Curry

Preparation time: *10 minutes*
Cooking time: *4 hours*
Servings: *6*
Ingredients:

- *Fresh ginger – 2 tbsp grated*
- *Garlic – 2 cloves, peeled and minced*
- *Cardamom – 2 tsp*
- *Onion – 1 peeled and hopped*
- *Cloves – 6*
- *Lamb meat – 1 pound, cubed*
- *Cumin powder – 2 tsp*
- *Garam masala – 1 tsp*
- *Chili powder – ½ tsp*
- *Turmeric – 1 tsp*
- *Coriander – 2 tsp*
- *Spinach – 1 pound*
- *Canned diced tomatoes – 14 ounces*

Directions:

In a slow cooker, mix lamb with tomatoes, spinach, ginger, garlic, onion, cardamom, cloves, cumin, garam masala, chili, turmeric, and coriander.

Stir well. Cover and cook on high for 4 hours.
Uncover slow cooker, stir the chili, divide into bowls, and serve.

Nutrition:
Calories 186 Total Fat 7.2g Saturated Fat 2.5g Cholesterol 38mg Sodium 477mg Total Carbohydrate 16.3g Dietary Fiber 5g Total Sugars 5g Protein 14.4g

14.Garlic Mushroom Frittata

Preparation time: *30 mins*
Cooking time: *10 to 30 mins*
Servings: *2*
Ingredients:

- *low-calorie cooking spray*
- *250g/9oz chestnut mushrooms, sliced*
- *1 small garlic clove, crushed*
- *1 tbsp thinly sliced fresh chives*
- *4 large free-range eggs, beaten*
- *freshly ground black pepper*
  For the salad
- *1 Little Gem lettuce, leaves separated*
- *100g/3½oz cherry tomatoes, halved*
- *1/3 cucumber, cut into chunks*

Directions*:*

Spray a small, flame-proof frying pan with oil and place over a high heat. (The base of the pan shouldn't be wider than about 18cm/7in.) Stir-fry the mushrooms in three batches for 2-3 minutes, or until softened and lightly browned. Tip the cooked mushrooms into a sieve over a bowl to catch any juices – you don't want the mushrooms to become soggy.

Return all the mushrooms to the pan and stir in the garlic and chives, and a pinch of ground black pepper. Cook for a further minute, then reduce the heat to low.

Preheat the grill to its hottest setting. Pour the eggs over the mushrooms. Cook for five minutes, or until almost set.

Place the pan under the grill for 3-4 minutes, or until set.

Combine the salad ingredients in a bowl.

Remove from the grill and loosen the sides of the frittata with a round-bladed knife. Turn out onto a board and cut into wedges. Serve hot or cold with the salad.

Nutrition:

243 kcal, 14g protein, 3.5g carbohydrate (of which 3g sugars), 14g fat (of which 4g saturates), 2.5g fiber and 0.6g salt per portion

15.Salmon BLT's

Preparation Time: *20 mins*
Cooking Time: *20 mins*
Servings: *4*
Ingredients:

- *8 slices bacon*
- *½ c. low-fat Greek yogurt*
- *¼ c. dill, chopped*
- *1 scallion, finely chopped*
- *1 tbsp. oil of choice*
- *4 oz. skinless salmon fillet*
- *1 tomato, sliced*
- *romaine lettuce for serving*
- *toasted bread for serving*
- *salt and pepper*

Directions:

Working in batches, cook bacon in a large skillet on medium heat until crisp for 5 to 6 minutes; transfer to a paper towel-lined plate.

Meanwhile, in a bowl, combine low-fat Greek yogurt, chopped dill, finely chopped scallion, and 1/4 tsp each salt and pepper.

Wipe out the skillet and heat 1 Tbsp oil on medium. Season four 4-oz pieces of skinless salmon fillet with ¼ tsp each salt and pepper and cook until opaque throughout, 1 to 2 minutes per side.

*Spread the yogurt mixture on 4 pieces of bread. Top with romaine lettuce, salmon, 1 sliced tomato, and bacon, then sandwich with another slice of bread. *

Nutrition:

485 calories, 42g protein, 43g carbs, 7g fiber, 10g sugars (6g added sugars), 15g fat (4g sat fat), 72mg cholesterol, 885mg sodium

16.Italian Style Meatballs With Courgette "Tagliatelle"

Preparation time: *30 mins*
Cooking time: *10 to 30 mins*
Servings: *2*
Ingredients:

For the meatballs

- *250g/9oz extra lean beef mince (5% fat or less)*
- *1 small onion, very finely chopped*
- *1 tsp dried mixed herbs*
- *calorie controlled cooking oil spray*
- *1 garlic clove, crushed*
- *227g/8oz can chopped tomatoes*
- *2 heaped tbsp finely shredded fresh basil leaves, plus extra to garnish*

For the courgette 'tagliatelle'

- *2 medium courgettes, trimmed and deseeded*
- *sea salt and freshly ground black pepper*

Directions:

Place the beef, half the onion, half the mixed herbs and a pinch of salt and pepper in a bowl and mix well. Form into 10 small balls.

Spray a medium non-stick frying pan with a little oil and cook the meatballs for 5-7 minutes, turning occasionally until browned on all sides. Transfer to a plate.

For the sauce, put the remaining onion in the same pan and cook over a low heat for three minutes, stirring. Add the garlic and cook for a few seconds.

Stir in the tomatoes, 300ml/10fl oz water, the remaining mixed herbs and shredded basil. Bring to the boil, stirring. Return the meatballs to the pan, reduce the heat to a simmer and cook for 20 minutes, stirring occasionally until the sauce is thick and the meatballs are cooked throughout.

Meanwhile, half-fill a medium pan with water and bring to the boil. Use a vegetable peeler to peel the courgettes into ribbons. Cook the courgette in the boiling water for one minute then drain.

Divide the courgette ribbons between two plates and top with the meatballs and sauce. Garnish with basil leaves.

Nutrition:
219 kcal per portion.

17.Red mullet with baked tomatoes

Preparation time: *30 mins*
Cooking time: *10 to 30 mins*
Servings: *4*
Ingredients:

For the tomatoes

- *375g/13oz mixed red and yellow cherry tomatoes*
- *320g/11½oz fine green beans, trimmed*
- *2 garlic cloves, finely chopped*
- *2 tbsp lemon juice*
- *low-calorie cooking spray*
- *salt and freshly ground black pepper*

For the red mullet

- *8 red mullet fillets, approximately 100g/3½oz each*
- *1 lemon, finely grated rind only*
- *2 tsp baby capers, drained*
- *2 spring onions, finely sliced*
- *To garnish*
- *2 tbsp chopped parsley*
- *8 caperberries*

Directions:
Preheat the oven to 200C/180C Fan/Gas 6.

Put the tomatoes in an ovenproof dish with the beans, garlic, lemon juice and spray with the oil. Season with salt and freshly ground black pepper and mix well. Bake for 10 minutes, or until the tomatoes and beans are tender.

Meanwhile, tear off 4 large sheets of foil and line with non-stick baking paper. Place 2 fish fillets on each piece of baking paper, then scatter over the lemon rind, capers and spring onions, season with salt and freshly ground black pepper. Fold over the paper-lined foil and scrunch the edges together to seal. Place the parcels on a large baking tray.

Place the fish parcels next to the vegetables in the oven and bake for a further 8-10 minutes, or until the flesh flakes easily when pressed in the centre with a knife.

Spoon the vegetables on to four serving plates and top each with two fish fillets. Garnish with the parsley and caperberries and serve.

Nutrition:
248 kcal.

18.Keto Crispy Ginger Mackerel Lunh Bowl

Preparation Time: *20 mins*
Cooking Time: *15 mins*
Servings: *2*
Ingredients:

Marinade:

- *1 tablespoon grated ginger*
- *1 tablespoon lemon juice*
- *3 tablespoons olive oil*
- *1 tablespoon coconut aminos*
- *Salt and pepper, to taste*

Lunch bowl:

- *2 (8-ounce) boneless mackerel fillets*
- *1-ounce almonds*
- *1 ½ cups broccoli*
- *1 tablespoon butter*
- *½ small yellow onion*
- *1/3 cup diced red bell pepper*
- *2 small sun-dried tomatoes, chopped*
- *4 tablespoons mashed avocado*

Directions:

Preheat the oven to 400 °F. Line a baking tray with parchment paper or foil. Mix together the grated ginger, lemon juice, olive oil, coconut aminos, and some salt and pepper. Rub half of the marinade on the mackerel fillets.

Lay the fillets onto the baking tray with the skin side facing up. Roast for 12-15 minutes or until the skin is crispy.

Spread the almonds out on a separate baking sheet. Roast for 5-6 minutes or until they brown. Take out of the oven and cool before chopping.

Lightly steam the broccoli until it's started to soften but isn't mushy. Roughly chop it up.

Preheat a pan over medium heat, then add the butter and allow it to melt. Fry the onions and peppers until they are soft.

Add the broccoli and sun-dried tomatoes, then continue cooking until warmed through.

Turn off the heat then mix in the rest of the dressing and roasted almonds. Serve with the avocado.

Nutrition:
649.55 Calories, 53.4g Fats, 9.2g Net Carbs, and 28.05g Protein

19.Zuppa Toscana with Cauliflower

Preparation time: *5 minutes*
Cooking time: *25 minutes*
Servings: *4*
Ingredients:

- *1-pound ground Italian sausage*
- *6 cups homemade low-sodium chicken stock*
- *2 cups cauliflower florets - 1 onion, finely chopped*
- *1 cup kale, stemmed and roughly chopped*
- *1 (14.5-ounce) can of full-fat coconut milk*
- *¼ teaspoon sea salt*
- *¼ teaspoon freshly cracked black pepper*

Directions:
On the Instant Pot, press "Sauté"and add the ground Italian sausage. Cook until brown, stirring occasionally and breaking up the meat with a wooden spoon.

Add the remaining ingredients except for the kale and coconut milk and stir until well combined.

Cover and cook for 10 minutes on high pressure. When done, release the pressure naturally and remove the lid. Stir in the kale and coconut milk. Cover and sit for 5 minutes or until the kale has wilted. Serve and enjoy!

Nutrition:
Calories 653 Carbohydrates 8g Protein 26g Fat 4g

20.Pork Carnitas

Preparation time: *20 minutes*
Cooking time: *1 hour*
Servings: *4*
Ingredients:

- *6 medium garlic cloves, minced*
- *2 teaspoons ground cumin*
- *1 teaspoon smoked paprika*
- *3 chipotle peppers in adobo sauce, minced*
- *1 teaspoon dried oregano*
- *2 bay leaves*
- *1 cup homemade low-sodium chicken broth*
- *Fine sea salt and freshly cracked black pepper*
- *2 tablespoons of olive oil*
- *2 ½ pounds boneless pork shoulder, cut into 4 large pieces*

Directions:

Season the pork shoulder with sea salt, black pepper, ground cumin, dried oregano, and smoked paprika.

On the Instant Pot, press "Sauté" and add the olive oil.

Once hot, add the pork pieces and sear for 4 minutes per side or until brown.

Add the remaining ingredients inside your Instant Pot. Cover and cook for 80 minutes on high pressure. When done, quick release the pressure and remove the lid.

Carefully shred the pork using two forks and continue to stir until well coated with the liquid.

Remove the bay leave and adjust the seasoning if necessary. Serve and enjoy!

Nutrition:
Calories 170 Carbohydrates 2g Protein 4g Fat 8g

Chapter 15

Snacks Recipes

21.Lamb and Flageolet Bean Stew

Preparation time: *30 mins*
Cooking time: *1 to 2 hours*
Servings: *4*
Ingredients:

- *1 tsp olive oil*
- *350g/12oz lean lamb, cubed*
- *16 pickling onions*
- *1 garlic clove, crushed*
- *600ml/20fl oz lamb stock (made with concentrated liquid stock)*
- *200g can of chopped tomatoes*
- *1 bouquet garni*
- *2 x 400g cans flageolet beans, drained and rinsed*
- *320g/11oz green beans*
- *250g/9oz cherry tomatoes*
- *freshly ground black pepper*

Directions:
Heat the oil in a flameproof casserole or saucepan, add the lamb and fry for 3-4 minutes until browned all over. Remove the lamb from the casserole and set aside.

Add the onions and garlic to the pan and fry for 4-5 minutes, or until the onions are beginning to brown.

Return the lamb and any juices to the pan. Add the stock, tomatoes, bouquet garni and beans. Bring to the boil, stirring, then cover and simmer for 1 hour, or until the lamb is just tender.

Meanwhile, bring a pan of water to the boil and blanch the green beans. Place in a bowl of ice-cold water.

Add the cherry tomatoes to the stew and season well with freshly ground black pepper. Continue to simmer for 10 minutes.

Divide the stew between four plates, place the green beans alongside and serve.

Nutrition:
288 kcal per portion

22.Chermoula Tofu and Roasted Vegetables

Preparation time: *30 mins*
Cooking time: *30 mins to 1 hour*
Servings: *4*
Ingredients:

For the chermoula tofu

- *25g/1oz coriander, finely chopped*
- *3 garlic cloves, chopped*
- *1 tsp cumin seeds, lightly crushed*
- *1 lemon, finely grated rind*
- *½ tsp dried crushed chillies*
- *1 tbsp olive oil*
- *250g/9oz tofu*

For the roasted vegetables

- *2 red onions, quartered*
- *2 courgettes, thickly sliced*
- *2 red peppers, deseeded and sliced*
- *2 yellow peppers, deseeded and sliced*
- *1 small aubergine, thickly sliced*
- *low-calorie cooking spray*
- *pinch salt*

Directions:

Preheat the oven to 200C/180C Fan/Gas 6.

For the chermoula, mix the coriander, garlic, cumin, lemon rind and chilies together with the oil and a little salt in a small bowl.

Pat the tofu dry on kitchen paper and cut it in half. Cut each half horizontally into thin slices. Spread the chermoula generously over the slices.

Scatter the vegetables in a roasting tin and spray with oil. Bake for about 45 minutes, until lightly browned, turning the ingredients once or twice during cooking.

Arrange the tofu slices over the vegetables, with the side spread with the chermoula uppermost, and bake for a further 10-15 minutes, or until the tofu is lightly coloured.

Divide the tofu and vegetables between four plates and serve.

Nutrition:
182 kcal per portion

23.Hearty Vegetable Soup

Preparation time: *30 mins*
Cooking time: *30 mins to 1 hour*
Servings: *2*
Ingredients:

- *calorie controlled cooking oil spray*
- *1 medium onion, sliced*
- *2 garlic cloves, thinly sliced*
- *2 celery sticks, trimmed and thinly sliced*
- *2 medium carrots or 2 yellow peppers, cut into 2cm/1in chunks*
- *400g/14oz tin chopped tomatoes*
- *1 vegetable stock cube*
- *1 tsp dried mixed herbs*
- *400g/14oz tin butter beans, drained and rinsed*
- *1 head young spring greens (approximately 125g/4½oz), trimmed and sliced*
- *sea salt and freshly ground black pepper*

Directions:
Spray a large non-stick saucepan with oil and cook the onion, garlic, celery and carrots or peppers gently for 10 minutes, stirring regularly until softened.

Add 750ml/26fl oz water and the chopped tomatoes. Crumble over the stock cube and stir in the dried herbs.
Bring to the boil, then reduce the heat to a simmer and

cook for 20 minutes.

Season the soup with salt and pepper and add the spring greens and butterbeans. Return to a gentle simmer and cook for a further 3-4 minutes or until the greens are softened. Season to taste and serve in deep bowls.

Nutrition:
219 kcal per portion.

24. Italian Omelet

Preparation Time: *10 mins*
Cooking Time: *20 mins*
Servings: *2*
Ingredients:

For Topping

- *1 medium (½ cup) tomato, seeded, chopped*
- *2 tablespoons sliced green onion*
- *1 tablespoon chopped fresh basil leaves*

For Eggs

- *1 tablespoon Land O Lakes® Butter*
- *1 teaspoon finely chopped fresh garlic*
- *4 large Land O Lakes® Eggs*
- *1 tablespoon water or milk*
- *¼ teaspoon salt*
- *1/8 teaspoon pepper*
- *½ cup shredded mozzarella cheese*
- *2 tablespoons shredded Parmesan cheese*

Directions:

Combine all topping ingredients in bowl; set aside.

Melt butter in 10-inch nonstick skillet over medium heat until sizzling. Add garlic; cook 1 minute.

Beat eggs, water, salt and pepper in bowl at low speed until light in color and well mixed. Pour eggs into hot skillet.

Cook 2 minutes; lift edge of eggs with heat proof spatula to allow uncooked portion to flow underneath 3-4 minutes or until mixture is almost set.

Sprinkle mozzarella cheese over half of omelet. Cover; let stand 1-2 minutes or until cheese is melted. Gently fold other half of omelet over cheese.

Place omelet onto plate; top with Parmesan cheese and tomato mixture. Cut in half.

Nutrition:
310 Calories 23 Fat (g) 455 Cholesterol (mg) 720 Sodium (mg) 4 Carbohydrates (g) 1 Dietary Fiber 21 Protein (g)

25.Chocolate Truffles

Preparation time: *10 minutes*
Cooking time: *60 minutes*
Servings: *12*
Ingredients:

- *Ripe Hass avocados – 2 pitted and skinned*
- *Coconut oil – 2 tbsp*
- *Premium cocoa powder – ½ cup*
- *Granulated sugar substitute – 1 tbsp*
- *Sugar free chocolate-flavored syrup – 2 tbsp*
- *Heavy whipping cream – 2 tbsp*
- *Bourbon – 2 tbsp*
- *Chopped pecans – ½ cup*

Directions:
Combine all ingredients except pecans in a small blender and process until smooth. Chill for 1 hour.

Make 1-inch balls and then roll in the pecans.

Chill in the refrigerator.

Nutrition:
Calories 124 Total Fat 11.7g Saturated Fat 4g Cholesterol 3mg Sodium 9mg Total Carbohydrate 4.5g Dietary Fiber 2.9g Total Sugars 0.4g Protein 1.8g

26.Blueberry Cake

Preparation time: *10 minutes*
Cooking time: *40 minutes*
Servings: *4*
Ingredients:

- *Almond flour - 2/3 cup*
- *Eggs – 5*
- *Almond milk – 1/3 cup*
- *Erythritol – ¼ cup*
- *Vanilla extract – 2 tsp*
- *Juice of 2 lemons*
- *Lemon zest – 1 tsp*
- *Baking soda – ½ tsp*
- *Pinch of salt*
- *Fresh blueberries – ½ cup*
- *Butter – 1 to 2 tbsp melted*
- *For the frosting:*
- *Heavy cream – ½ cup*
- *Juice of 1 lemon*
- *Erythritol– 1/8 cup*

Directions:
Preheat the oven to 350°F.

In a bowl, add the almond flour, eggs, and almond milk and mix well until smooth.

Then add the erythritol, a pinch of salt, baking soda, lemon zest, lemon juice, and vanilla extract. Mix and combine well.

Fold in the blueberries.

Use the butter to grease the springform pans.

Pour the batter into the two greased pans.

Place on a baking sheet for even baking.

Place in the oven to bake until cooked through in the middle and slightly brown on the top about 35 to 40 minutes.

Allow to cool before removing from the pan.

Mix together the erythritol, lemon juice, heavy cream for the frosting. Mix well.

Pour frosting on top and spread. Serve.

Nutrition:
Calories 272 Total Fat 23.8g Saturated Fat 13.2g Cholesterol 240mg Sodium 287mg Total Carbohydrate 21g Dietary Fiber 1.4g Total Sugars 18.2g Protein 8.9g

27.Low-Carb Brownies

Preparation time: *10 minutes*
Cooking time: *20 minutes*
Servings: *16*
Ingredients:

- *7 tablespoons Coconut oil, melted*
- *6 tablespoons Plant-Based sweetener*
- *1 Large egg*
- *2 Egg yolk*
- *1/2 tsp Mint extract*
- *5 ounces Sugar-free dark chocolate*
- *¼ cup Plant-based chocolate protein powder*
- *1 tsp Baking soda*
- *¼ tsp Sea salt*
- *2 tablespoons vanilla almond milk, Unsweetened*

Directions:
Start by preheating the oven to 350°F and then take an 8x8 inch pan and line it with parchment paper, being sure to leave some extra sticking up to use later to help you get them out of the pan after they are cooked.

Into a medium-sized vessel, use a hand mixer, and blend 5 Tablespoons of the coconut oil (save the rest for later), as well as the egg, Erythritol, egg yolks, and the mint extract all together for 1 minute. After this minute, the mixture will become a lighter yellow hue.

Take 4 oz of the chocolate and put it in a (microwave-safe) bowl, as well as with the other 2 Tablespoons of melted coconut oil.

Cook this chocolate and oil mixture on half power, at 30-second intervals, being sure to stir at each interval, just until the chocolate becomes melted and smooth

While the egg mixture is being beaten, add in the melted chocolate mixture into the egg mixture until this becomes thick and homogenous.

Add in your protein powder of choice, salt, baking soda, and stir until homogenous. Then, vigorously whisk your almond milk in until the batter becomes a bit smoother.

Finely chop the rest of your chocolate and stir these bits of chocolate into the batter you have made.

Spread the batter evenly into the pan you have prepared, and bake this until the edges of the batter just begin to become darker, and the center of the batter rises a little bit. You can also tell by sliding a toothpick into the middle, and when it comes out clean, it is ready. This will take approximately 20 to 21 minutes. Be sure that you do NOT over bake them!

Let them cool in the pan they cooked in for about 20 minutes. Then, carefully use the excess paper handles to take the brownies out of the pan and put them onto a wire cooling rack.

Make sure that they cool completely, and when they do, cut them, and they are ready to eat!

Nutrition:
Calories 107 Fats 10g Carbohydrates 5.7g Protein 2.5g

28.Apple Bread

Preparation time: *10 minutes*
Cooking time: *20 minutes*
Servings: *10*
Ingredients:

- *½ cup honey*
- *½ tsp. nutmeg*
- *½ tsp. salt*
- *1 cup applesauce, sweetened*
- *1 tsp. baking soda*
- *1 tsp. vanilla extract*
- *2 ¼ cup whole wheat flour*
- *2 large eggs*
- *2 tbsp. vegetable oil*
- *2 tsp. baking powder*
- *2 tsp. cinnamon*
- *4 cup apples, diced*

Directions:

Preheat oven to 375° Fahrenheit and oil a loaf pan with non-stick spray or your choice of oil.

Beat eggs in a mixing bowl and stir until completely smooth.

Add the honey, oil, applesauce, cinnamon, vanilla, nutmeg, baking powder, baking soda, and salt. Whisk until completely combined and smooth.

Add the flour into the bowl and whisk to combine, making sure not to over-mix. Simply stir it enough to incorporate the flour.

Add apples to the batter and mix once more to combine.

Pour the batter into the loaf pan and smooth the top with your spatula.

Bake for 60 minutes, or until an inserted toothpick in the center comes out clean.

Let stand for 10 minutes, then transfer the loaf to a cooling rack to cool completely.

Slice into 10 pieces and serve!

Nutrition:
Calories 210 Carbohydrates 41g Fats 5g Protein 5g

29.Coconut Protein Balls

Preparation time: *20 minutes*
Cooking time: *0 minutes*
Servings: *27*
Ingredients:

- *¼ cup dark chocolate chips*
- *½ cup coconut flakes, unsweetened*
- *½ cup water*
- *1 ½ cup almonds, raw & unsalted*
- *2 tbsp. cocoa powder, unsweetened*
- *3 cup Medjool dates, pitted*
- *4 scoops whey protein powder, unsweetened*

Directions:
Blend almonds in a food processor until a flour is formed. Add the water and dates to the flour and continue to process until fully combined. You may need to stop intermittently to scrape down the sides of the bowl.

Add cocoa and protein to the processor and continue to process until well combined. You may need to stop intermittently to scrape down the sides of the bowl.

Pull the blade out of the processor (carefully!) and use your spatula to gather all of the dough in one place inside the processor container.

On a plate or in a large, shallow dish, spread the coconut flakes.

Scoop out a little bit of the dough at a time using a spoon, and roll it into balls, then roll each one in the coconut flakes.

Refrigerate for at least 30 min before enjoying.

Nutrition:
Calories 108 Carbohydrates 16g Fats 4g   Protein 5g

30.Chocolate Chia Pudding

Preparation time: *3 minutes*
Cooking time: *0 minutes*
Servings: *1*
Ingredients:

- *¾ cup milk, unsweetened*
- *2 tsp. honey*
- *1 tsp. vanilla extract*
- *4 tbsp. chia seeds*
- *1 tbsp. cocoa powder, unsweetened*

Directions:
In a glass jar or container, combine all liquid ingredients and mix completely.

Add chia seeds and cocoa powder and mix completely.

Allow everything to sit for about 10 minutes before stirring once again, then sealing tightly and storing in the refrigerator overnight.

Stir well before eating and enjoy cold!

Nutrition:
Calories 329 Carbohydrates 40g Fats 14g Protein 14g

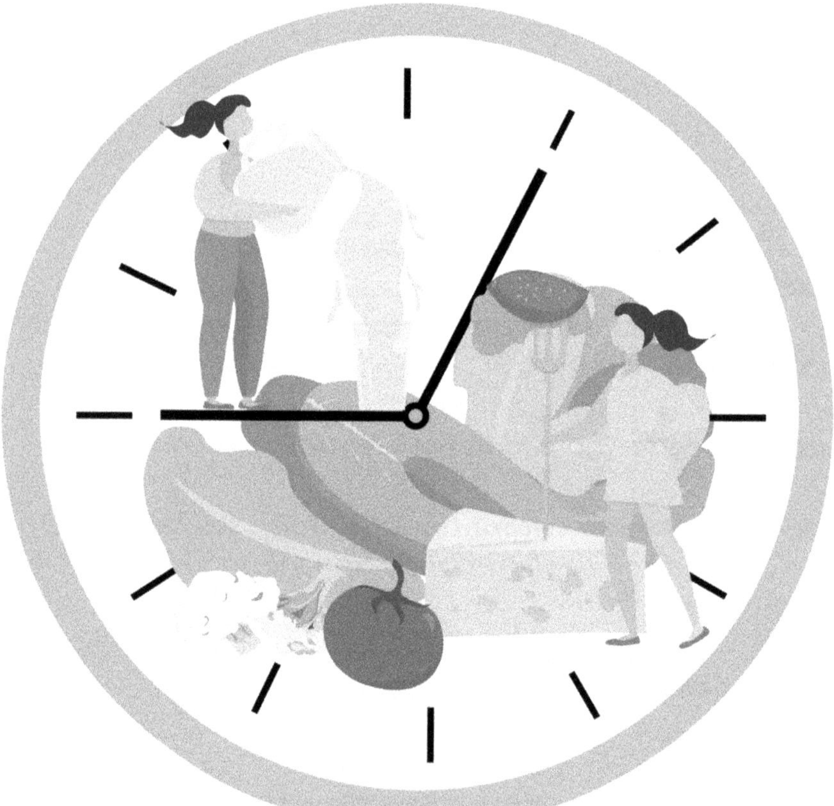

Conclusion

In anything new that we try, there is a chance that we may fall off track. Fasting or following a new diet plan are no different. The focus should not be on the fact that you fell off but on how you decide to come back and approach it again. You need not give up altogether if you have a day or two where you did not accomplish your full fast. You just need to re-examine your plan and approach it in a different way. Maybe your fasting period was too long for your first try. Maybe your fasting and eating windows did not match up with your sleep-wake cycle as well as they could have. Any of these factors can be adjusted to better suit your lifestyle needs and make fasting or a specific diet work for you. Being able to be flexible with yourself is something that is trying a new diet regimen like this can teach you. With the human body, there is never a right or a wrong way to approach anything; there is only a multitude of different ways and some that will be better for your specific body and mind than others. Being open to trying different variations and adjusting your plan as you go can be the difference between success and deciding to give up.

Intermittent fasting can be very challenging at first but if you can get over the few times and stick to it, it is immensely rewarding.

Don't give up if you feel that the fasting plan you have chosen is too much for you. Ask your medical advisor to help you either modify your current plan or try another one. Not everyone is suited to each plan. You may find you need to try one or two before you are comfortable.

If you fall off track, scale your plan back a little bit and try it again. If you are worried that you are not doing enough, begin with the scaled back plan, and get used to this first, you can always increase your fasting times later on once you know you are completely comfortable with a shorter fasting time.

If this book has taught you anything, the hope is that it has taught you how many variables are involved when it comes to health and wellness. This book aimed to share with you the plethora of options that are available to you when it comes to autophagy and inducing it within the cells of your body.
Think back on the many options that were laid out for you involving diet options and specific foods that have the ability to induce autophagy in the brain. It is your job now to decide which of these foods or supplements to include in your life and to practice a sort of trial and error, noting which ones make you feel great and which ones you prefer to go without. With all of this information, you can decide which ways fit best with your specific lifestyle and your preferences.

As you take all of this information forth with you, it may seem overwhelming to begin applying this into your own life. Remember, life is a process, and you do not need to expect perfection from yourself. By taking the steps to read this book, you are already on your way to changing your life.

Lightning Source UK Ltd.
Milton Keynes UK
...0250221120
...78

9 781914 036125